SPARTANAT
BLACK BOOK

2

SPARTANAT

spartanat.com

TACTICAL MEDICINE

LIFESAVING IS A MATTER OF MINUTES

TCCC—THE BASICS OF CASUALTY CARE

CARSTEN DOMBROWSKI

TABLE OF CONTENTS

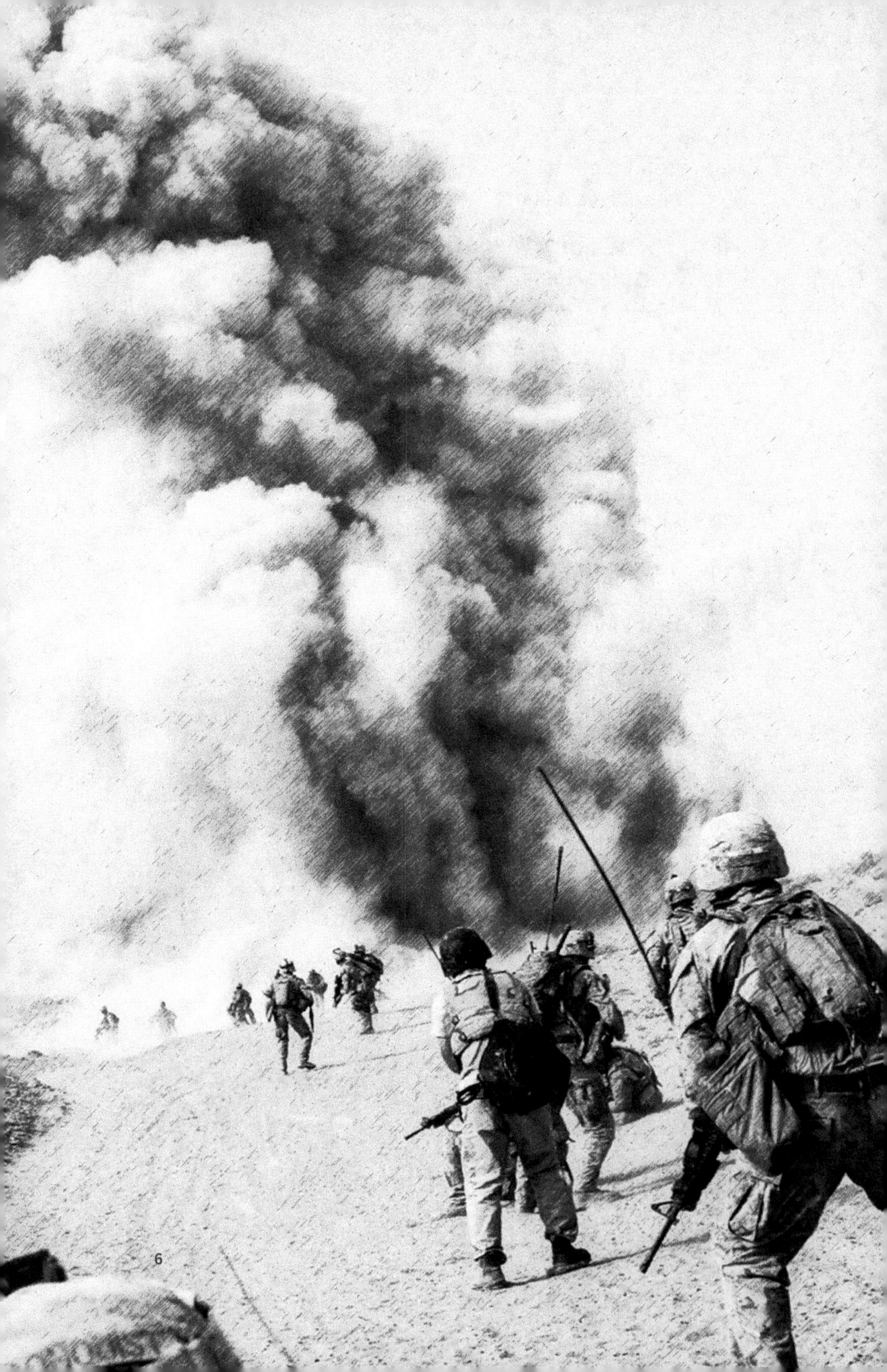

INTRODUCTION:
GOOD MEDICINE IN BAD PLACES

"TACTICAL MEDICINE" IS A COLLECTIVE TERM FOR MEDICINE OUTSIDE THE COMFORT ZONE, UNDER WHICH MANY TERMS AND CARE CONCEPTS CAN BE CATEGORIZED, BE IT WILDERNESS, REMOTE, COMBAT, OPERATIONAL, OR WHICHEVER OTHER MEDICINE.

Tactical Medicine and its subgroups have a few key characteristics that distinguish them from individual medicine.

Firstly, tactics determine the procedure for treating patients in Tactical Medicine. In other words, the mission comes before providing care or preventing danger. This is often very strange for people foreign to this philosophy. Slogans like "The best medicine on the battlefield is fire superiority" show very clearly what this means.

Furthermore, limited material or personnel resources and extended rescue routes characterize Tactical Medicine's working conditions.

These necessitate completely different procedures or the use of special materials that are rarely used by regular rescue services.

Tactical Medicine is no competitor to standard medicine. It is a supplement to the supply chain in situations where the regular rescue services are temporarily overwhelmed by a threat situation or only able to arrive much later due to long rescue chains.

This book is intended to help you classify terms correctly and understand the basics of Tactical Medicine more easily, so that you can handle the subject practically. The book itself will not create tactical medics or authentic-looking instructors. Whoever has not yet mastered the individual techniques, lacks the so-called "skills", and has no overall understanding of Tactical Medicine concerns should not consider themselves familiar with this field of work.

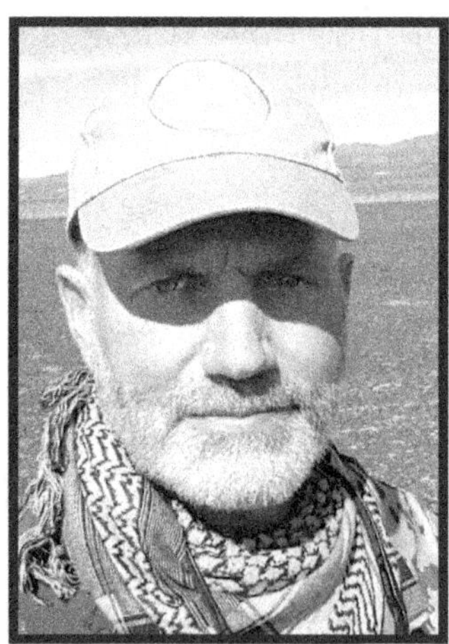

Carsten Dombrowski

CAUTION:

READING THIS BOOK ALONE WILL NOT STOP A BLEEDING!

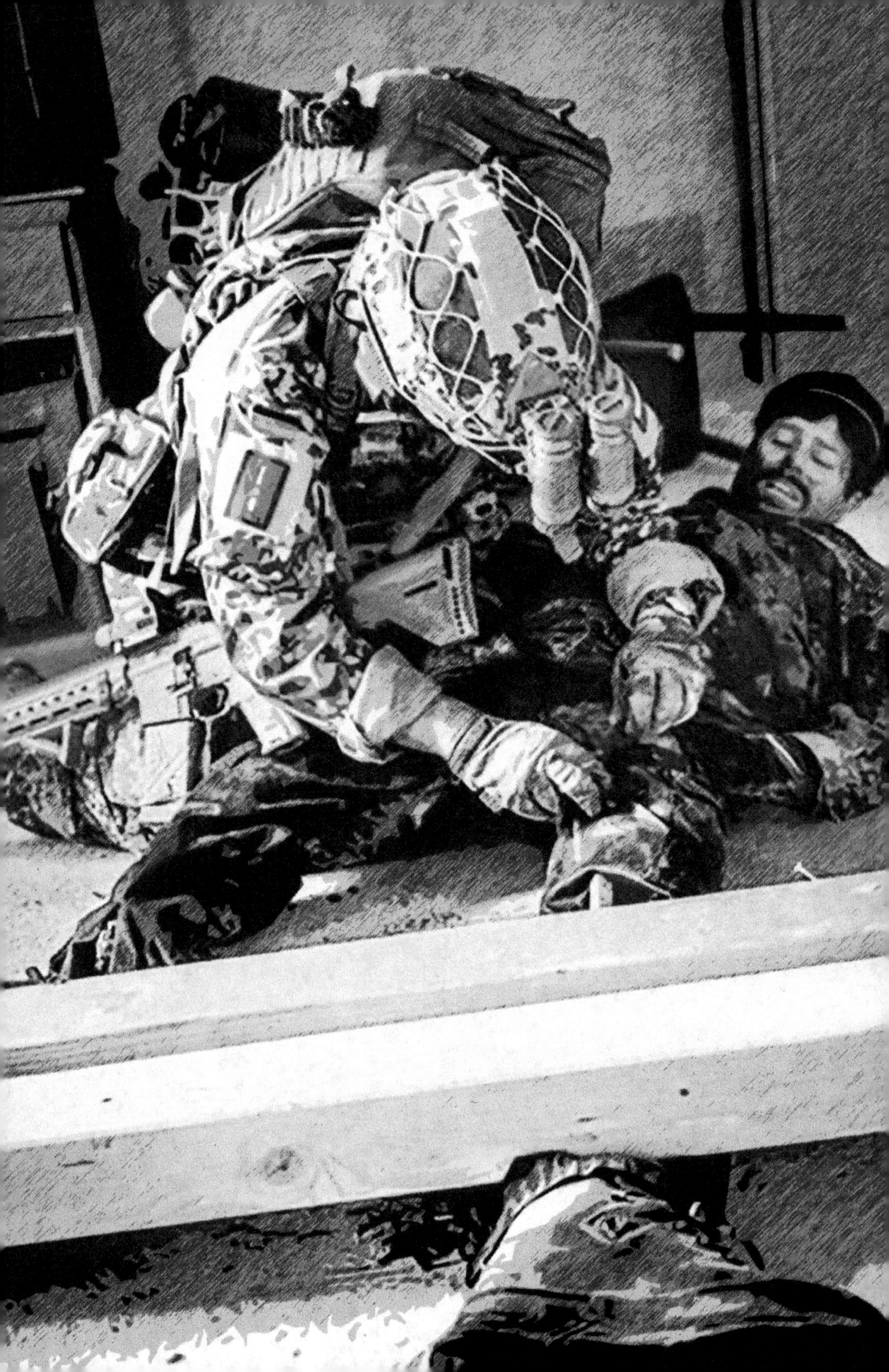

TACTICAL MEDICINE: A HISTORY

FROM THE WORLD WARS TO VIETNAM

There was medical care for the wounded on the battlefield and in field hospitals in the wars or armed conflicts of the past as well, of course. There was also a form of qualified transport of the wounded. Nevertheless, the high casualty figures of those wars cannot be explained solely by the massive firepower of weapons or the conflicts' duration. Medical care as well as tactical operational capabilities were far removed from what is standard today (see Chapter 3 for more detail). Here I just want to briefly mention the introduction of **Forward Air Medevac**, employed by the U.S. **Dustoff** rescue operations to pick up the wounded directly off the jungle battlefield during the Vietnam war. This innovative use of helicopters for tactical casualty transport reduced the time it took for a wounded person to receive medical treatment substantially. This certainly contributed to a better chance of survival (more on this in Chapter 16).

MOGADISHU AND TCCC

Operation "Gothic Serpent" and the resulting battle in Mogadishu (Somalia) on October 4, 1993, set the course for casualty care. Even though few U.S. soldiers were killed—at least compared to battles on the Western Front or in the Pacific theater during World War II—the experience and its analysis led to a massive change of heart among U.S. military staff. That was the birth of **Tactical Combat Casualty Care**, or **TCCC** for short.

AFGHANISTAN AND MODERN TIMES

With post-9/11 events, the areas of U.S., German, and other armed forces' deployment increased significantly. The Balkans mission in the late 1990s and especially Afghanistan indicated, particularly to the German Federal Armed Forces (Bundeswehr), that in terms of medical service concepts, many things had to be realigned. After the heavy fighting of 2010, debate about the benefits of new first aid materials finally stopped. For operational reasons, the Bundeswehr had arrived at Tactical Medicine. In those days, the casualty figures no longer allowed for any other option or way of thinking.

TACTICAL COMBAT CASUALTY CARE

TCCC

THE WHO'S WHO OF TACTICAL MEDICINE

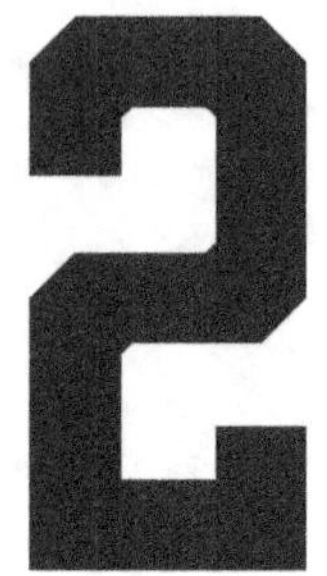

IN ORDER TO BETTER UNDERSTAND CONTEXTS OR CIRCUMSTANCES, IT IS HELPFUL TO KNOW NAMES AND ABBREVIATIONS FROM THE SPECTRUM OF TACTICAL MEDICINE.

This includes people as well as institutions that have rendered outstanding services to Tactical Medicine.

▶ **Frank Butler** is the best-known of all personalities when it comes to naming the greats of Tactical Medicine. As a doctor and member of the Navy SEALs, he and **John Hagmann** made the decisive proposals that led to the TCCC (Tactical Combat Casualty Care) concept. Butler also worked for the TCCC Committee for many years. Hagmann accompanied him in this work for a long time, but due to internal U.S. incidences, he can no longer be quoted today, or only to a limited extent.

▶ **THE TCCC Committee**, or coTCCC for short, is a leadership and development forum for the TCCC cause. Consisting of 42 permanent voting members from all branches of the U.S. armed forces and the U.S. Coast Guard, coTCCC works with numerous national and international working groups. It is also in constant dialogue with civil institutions for trauma care. It is responsible for annually updating the **TCCC Guidelines**. These guidelines serve as the legitimate basis for the protocols of many organizations and specialist areas involved in this field worldwide.

gu.usa.gov/xUfxT

▶ **The TECC Committee** (Tactical Emergency Casualty Care) is the civilian counterpart to coTCCC and has developed from civilian institutions adapting to the overall topic of Tactical Medicine. The training of the police and other security authorities was organized and brought together under the TECC umbrella. For the target group of Law Enforcement Officers and Operators (LEO), this has become necessary due to the global terrorist threat situation. **c-tecc.org**

▶ **NAEMT** (National Association of Emergency Medical Technicians) has set itself the task of standardizing global preclinical education and training. Through its own certified "School Houses," it offers many medical courses, including on the concepts of TCCC and TECC. **naemt.org**

▶ In 2008, **TREMA** (Tactical Rescue Emergency Medical Association) was founded in response to the need to introduce Tactical Medicine to the German Federal Armed Forces and police special forces. Founded as a registered association to better bundle their interests, TREMA quickly grew into a specialist association for Tactical Medicine across the German-speaking countries. To this day, the TREMA Guidelines serve as a citable counterpart to the TCCC Guidelines.

tremaonline.info

▶ Globally, there are two leading specialist conferences on Tactical Medicine. These are **SOMA** (Special Operations Medical Association) in the U.S. and **CMC** (Combat Medical Conference) in Germany, alternating with France since 2022. With well over 1,400 visitors, these two events are unique, even though there are smaller conferences of equal quality in Germany and abroad as well.

specialoperationmedicine.org
cmc-conference.de

TACTICAL MEDICINE: STATISTICAL FOUNDATIONS

3

CAUSES OF DEATH ON THE BATTLEFIELD AND THE THREE TYPES OF CASUALTIES

Based on the analyses of past wars and their military casualty figures—focusing on the Korea and Vietnam wars, the Iraq wars, and Afghanistan—sober observations revealed that a considerable number of moribund or actually KIA soldiers on the battlefield would not have had to die if the right Tactical Medicine measures had been applied at the right time.

**THE ANALYSES REVEALED THREE
MAIN GROUPS OF POTENTIAL CAUSES OF DEATH:**

— **9% bleeding to death from extremity injuries,**
— **5% penetrating thoracic injuries,**
— **1% airway obstruction.**

A closer look at all medical measures within Tactical Medicine focuses on the 14% of wounded who, without adequate initial medical care, die on the battlefield. These figures are from the first years of the study and certainly require a renewed analysis, as many things have developed since then.

Despite all measures, there will always be the following three groups of wounded:

1. WOUNDED WHO DIE, NO MATTER WHAT WE DO FOR THEM,

2. WOUNDED WHO SURVIVE, NO MATTER WHAT WE DO FOR THEM,

3. WOUNDED WHO SURVIVE IF WE DO THE RIGHT THING AT THE RIGHT TIME.

WHY DO PATIENTS SURVIVE THESE DAYS?

In addition to the introduction of TCCC, a whole host of other changes have contributed to the permanent casualty reduction on the battlefield in recent years. There have been tactical, but also organizational, measures worth mentioning here:

- ▶ **Improved equipment for soldiers with the introduction of ballistic protective equipment,**

- ▶ **improvement of medical first-aid training in accordance with the TCCC and TECC concepts;**

- ▶ **introduction and use of primarily airborne rescue vessels (such as helicopters) to shorten transport times and skip intermediate medical levels,**

- ▶ **introduction and use of protected medical transport vehicles,**

- ▶ **use of Forward Surgery Teams with combat surgery capacity up to Surgery Damage Control.**

THE "GOLDEN HOUR" OR "PLATINUM FIVE MINUTES" ILLUSTRATE HOW THE FIRST RESPONDER'S ROLE ESSENTIALLY CONTRIBUTES TO WHETHER A WOUNDED PERSON—WITH MASSIVE BLEEDING FROM THE EXTREMITIES, FOR EXAMPLE— SURVIVES OR NOT.

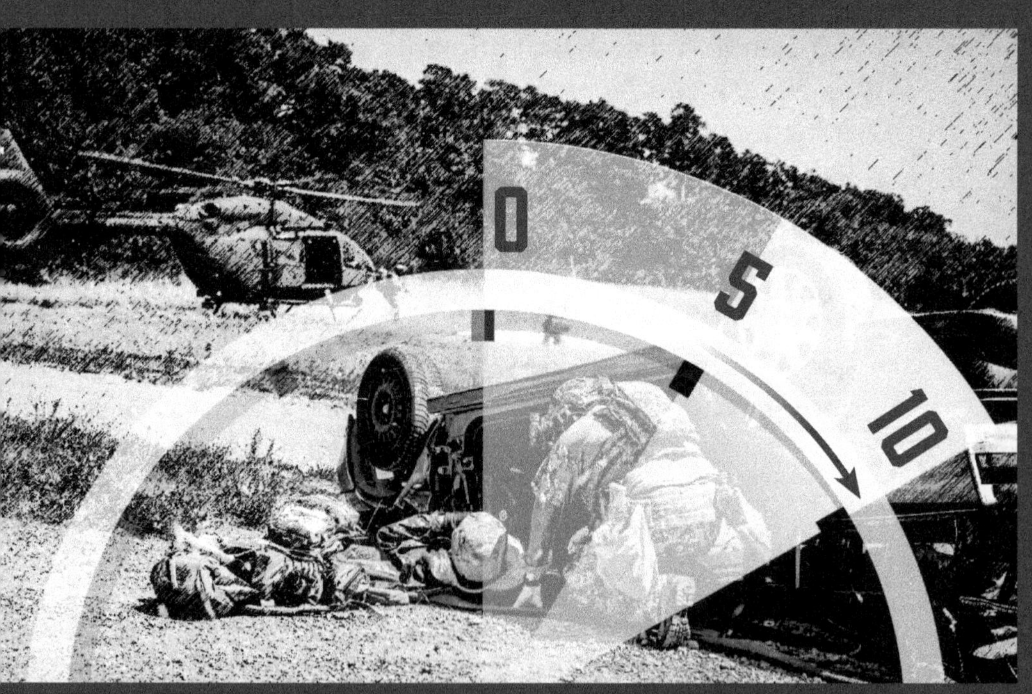

THE ZONE MODEL OF TACTICAL MEDICINE 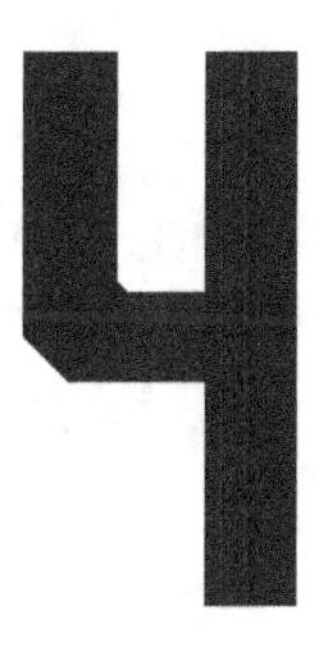

Regardless of which Tactical Medicine concept is used, in principle, all areas work with the so-called zone model. The following is an overview for better understanding and comparison. In application, it is irrelevant which of the options presented here a rescuer chooses. However, it is important to understand the need to adapt to the tactical situation. Professional paramedics, in particular, tend to focus exclusively on the patient and initially ignore the general on-site situation.

TCCC	Care Under Fire	Tactical Field Care	Tactical Evacuation Care
TECC	Direct Threat Care	Indirect Threat Care	Evacuation Care
OTHER	Red Zone	Yellow Zone	Green Zone
	Unsafe Zone	Partially Safe Zone	Safe Zone

▶ CARE UNDER FIRE IS THE PHASE IN WHICH THERE IS IMMEDIATE DANGER TO THE LIVES OF THE WOUNDED BUT ALSO TO THE HELPERS.

Medical measures should be reduced to the absolute minimum. From a medical point of view, the most that can be done is to stop the bleeding, e.g., by using a tourniquet. As part of further procedures, a decision must then be made whether the threat can be eliminated or minimized or whether an evacuation must be carried out in order to rescue the victim from the danger zone. The term **"crash rescue"** is used here, meaning that proper, careful patient transport is abandoned in favor of quick delivery to reduce the danger.

▶ TACTICAL FIELD CARE ENABLES AN INITIAL MEDICAL EXAMINATION ACCORDING TO AN EXAMINATION SCHEME OR INITIAL CARE BEYOND LIFE-SAVING MEASURES.

In this phase, enemy pressure has been relieved, dangers have been reduced, or the casualty has been evacuated from the danger zone. In addition to treatment, tactical decisions continue to be made in this phase. For example, an extended reporting scheme is sent out, such as the 9 Line Medevac Request (see Chapter 12). Close cooperation between the medical care and security teams is now important, as the situation could escalate again at any time and result in a further change in the team's position. For this reason, medical forces are urged to prepare themselves and the wounded for evacuation at all times and not to fall into "peacetime medicine" mode. In concrete terms, this means working from the medical kit bags to avoid losing medical supplies in the event of a sudden change of situation.

▶ TACTICAL EVACUATION CARE IS THE THIRD AND LAST TCCC PHASE. HERE, CRITICAL TACTICAL-SURGICAL MEASURES HAVE ALREADY BEEN INITIATED.

The patient is fit for transport, care for the needed transportation times and means of transport have been procured, and medical measures carried out have been documented. Despite relative situational safety, this phase can still get heated. In the past, especially approaching rescue helicopters have repeatedly attracted heavy enemy fire, or the distance to a landing zone has been underestimated by ground forces, resulting in evacuation forces taking over casualties being avoidably hampered. The establishment of a helicopter landing zone by securing forces is also an activity that needs to be practiced repeatedly.

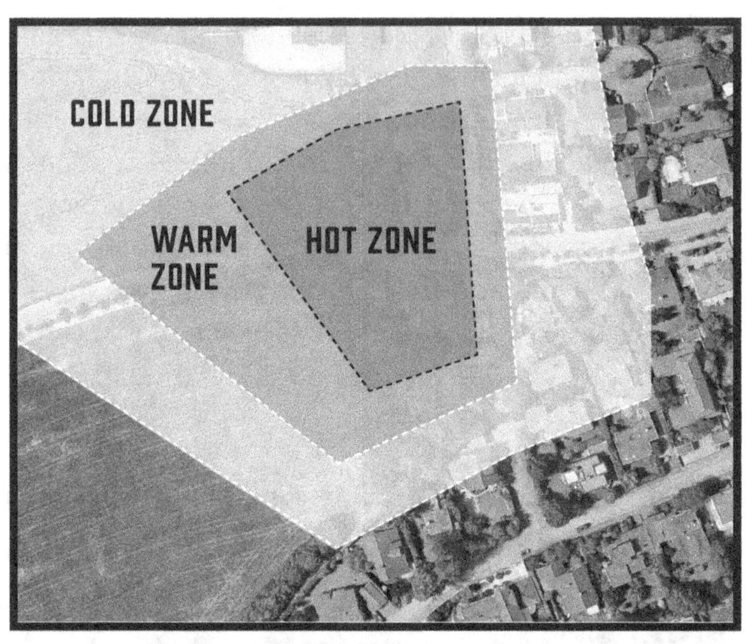

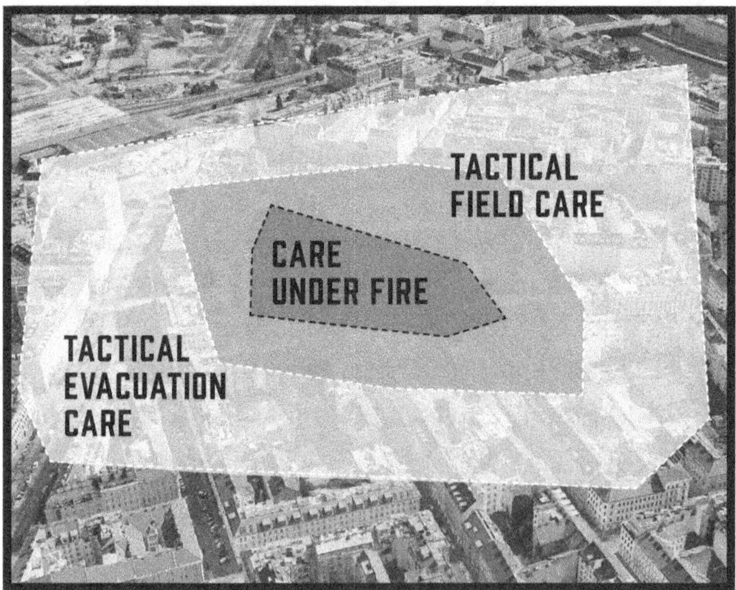

The danger determines the zone. This, in turn, determines what is possible for helpers.

SUMMARY:

As the slogan "<u>Good medicine in bad places</u>" suggests, there are situations in which extensive medical measures and treatments are inappropriate. <u>Assessing the safety situation</u> and <u>responding</u> to it is the <u>top priority</u> in Tactical Medicine. All too often, aid workers have put themselves and their wounded in dangerous situations because they did not follow the zone model. In some cases, it is already of great help to guide a wounded man in applying a tourniquet from one's own cover.

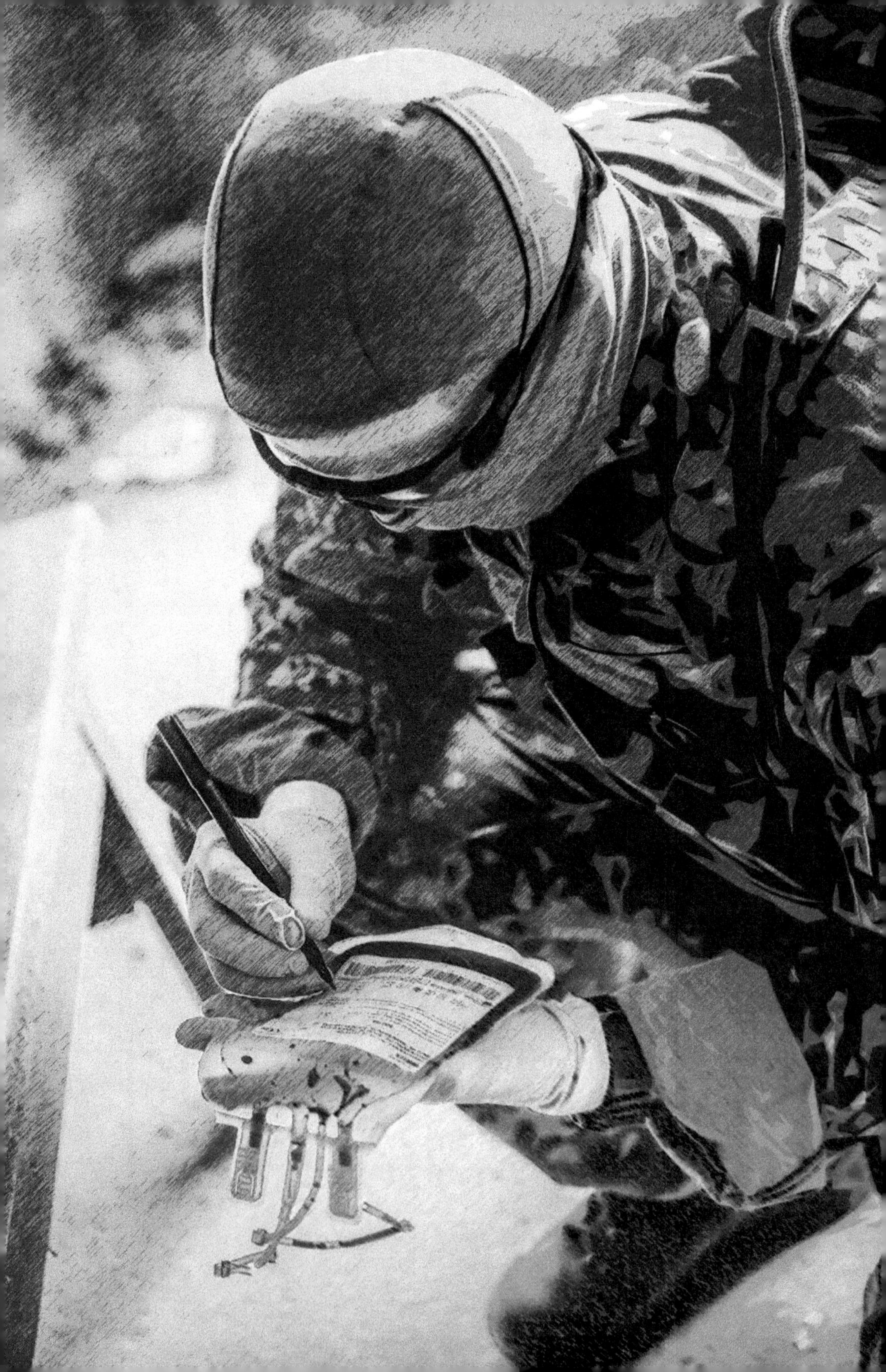

EXAMINATION SCHEMES 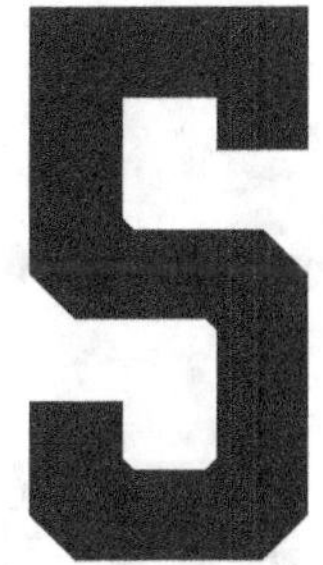

THERE ARE NOW SEVERAL SCHEMES FOR EXAMINING A CASUALTY IN THE TACTICAL FIELD CARE PHASE.

The **MARCH** approach is used in both the **TCCC** and **TECC concepts.** The two most common variants are compared below. Both have their areas of application and legitimacy.

However, before an injured person is examined, the overall situation must also be assessed according to a scheme. This is helpful in determining self-protection as well as the initial factors of the injury mechanism.

The following is an overview for better understanding and comparison. In application, it is irrelevant which of the options presented here a rescuer follows.

SICK:

An initial assessment of whether the immediate area is safe. This can include many aspects: collapsing buildings, fires, leaking liquids, threatening animals, and many more. Based on this, the rescuer decides whether they can minimize the danger or, if necessary, evacuate the injured person from the area.

The identification of things that could influence care or could have triggered the situation. Objects lying around, the overall impression of a location, people standing around, or other aspects that are immediately conspicuous are assessed visually or through other sensory organs by the rescuer. A strong smell of gas would be a good example.

CRITICAL
CBLEEDING

This is the type of bleeding that can be recognized immediately by the first arriving rescuer without touching the patient, solely on the basis of heavy bleeding or pools of blood that have already formed. Bleeding should be the first focus of the rescuers' attention.

KINE-
KMATICS

This is a generic term for the energy that may have affected the injured person or may have led to the injury. Fall height or vehicle involvement with deployed airbags would be relevant indications. It is sometimes helpful to ask witnesses whether they can provide any information on this.

Now that the SICK pattern has been recorded, the first physical contact with the patient is made. If the safety situation permits, the examination begins according to the following schemes:

MARCH/CABCD/E:

MASSIVE BLEE-DING	Quickly **frisk the major sources of bleeding**, such as the neck, armpit, groin, legs, and arms (the so-called rapid blood sweep).	**C** Critical bleeding
AIR-WAYS	Address the patient, look into the mouth, remove foreign bodies if necessary, and extend the head. Then check for breathing: hear, see, and feel. If the patient is unconscious, an **airway can already be secured** using NPA.	**A** Airways
RESPI-RATION	In order to assess the **quality of breathing** and check for injuries to the chest, it is examined for bruises, hematomas, injuries, and stability. The back and the armpit area should also be examined very carefully. Penetrating injuries are now taped, e.g., using a chest seal.	**B** Breathing

CIRCU-LATION	In order to **assess the circulatory situation** of the injured person, the pulses on the wrist and neck are felt first. If a pulse is found at the wrist, the blood pressure values are still stable. Counting to determine the pulse quality is postponed. After the pulses, all four extremities are examined for injuries and stability. The abdomen and pelvis are also examined for signs of injury. Bruises, misalignment, or similar signs can be detected during this examination.	**C** **Circulation**
HEAD **A**ND **HEAT**	As a final examination measure, the patient's **head is examined**. This involves looking into all the head orifices. The ears and nose are examined for bleeding, the mouth for tongue bites and signs of fracture, and the eyes for neurological deficits, which can be recognized by the pupillary reaction. The scheme used as an aid for pupil reaction is **PERRLA**: The **p**upils should be **e**qual, **r**ound, and **r**eact to **l**ight and **a**ccommodation. **Heat conservation** is optimized, and **documentation** is started in this phase.	**D/E** **Disability/ Exposure**

MEDIC EQUIPMENT / MARCH SYSTEM

MASSIVE BLEEDING. Primarily materials for hemostasis, but also for wound care. This includes various tourniquets—in this specific case, CAT Generation 7 and SWAT. In addition, there are elastic wound dressings, hemostatic agents, gauze bandages, and compresses. Also, materials for wound treatment, such as bandage scissors, triangular cloths, tape, and plaster sets. There is a pelvic sling on the upper edge to immobilize a possible pelvic fracture.

AIRWAYS AND RESPIRATION. This includes not only breathing itself, but also the entire airway and respiratory system. The associated materials are therefore also shown here. The well-known Wendl tubes, various chest seals, and several chest puncture needles for tension pneumothorax are among the materials required to treat A and R problems.

CIRCULATION / HEAD AND HEAT. These materials are used to stabilize circulation and combat cooling: infusion solutions with corresponding venous cannulas, splints for fixing and immobilizing extremities in the event of fractures, and various materials for heat retention. A chemical warming blanket for active warming can also be seen here.

The medic depicted has also laid out personal protective equipment and additional gear, such as his weapon and magazines.

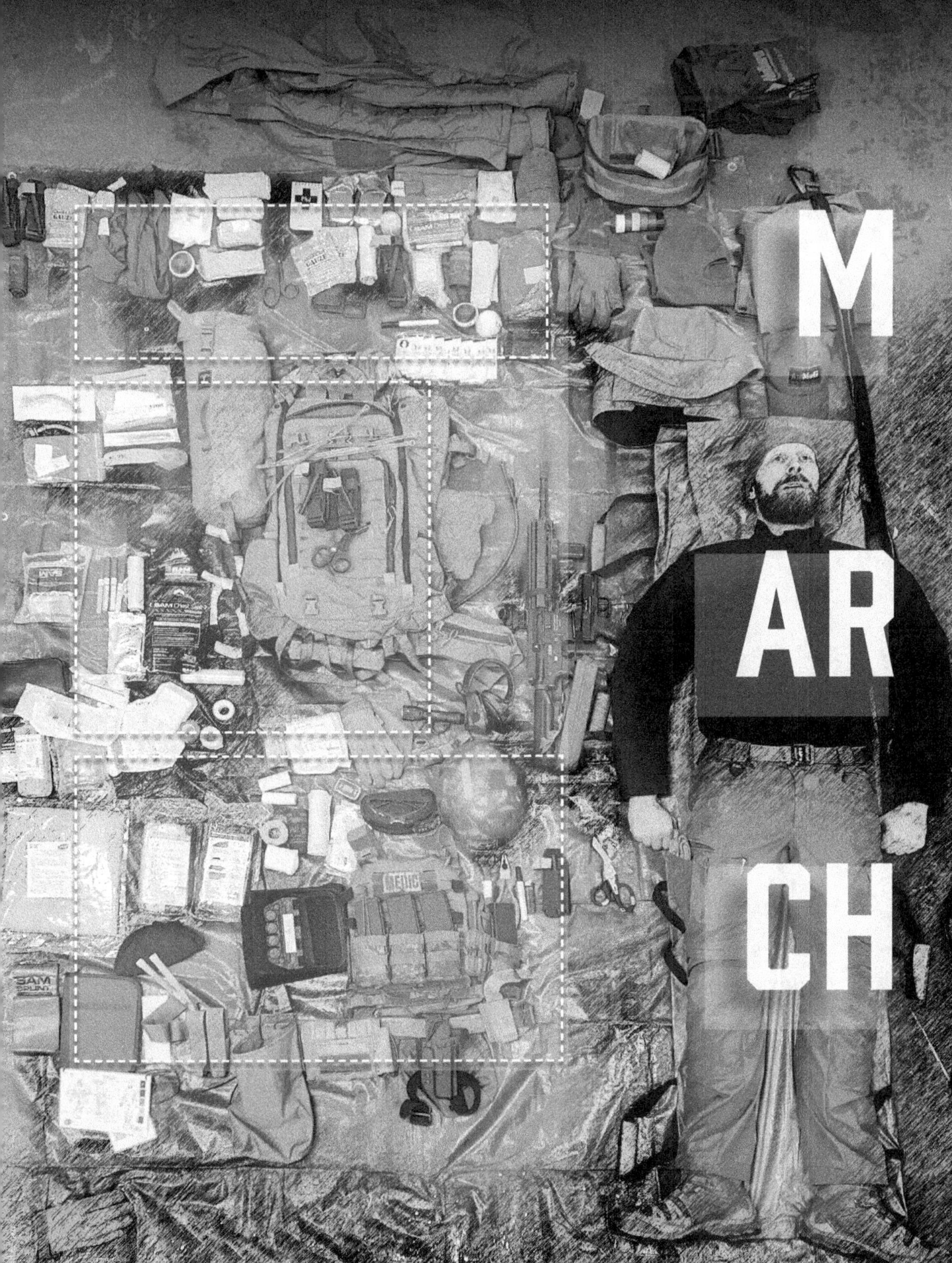
M
AR
CH

Once the investigation has been completed according to one of the schemes above, all life-threatening problems should have been preliminarily treated **(<u>Treat first what kills first</u>)** and an overall impression should have been gained.

The latter is communicated to the tactical leader on site. At the same time, it is asked how much time is left for further treatment. This is a matter of close cooperation between the elements of security and those of medical assistance, again. **<u>Tactics determine medicine!</u>**

SUMMARY:
It is close to irrelevant which scheme is used when examining the patient. It is important that all life-threatening issues are recognized and treated immediately. Everything else is then determined by good cooperation between helpers and tactical elements. Self-protection always comes first.

HEMOSTASIS 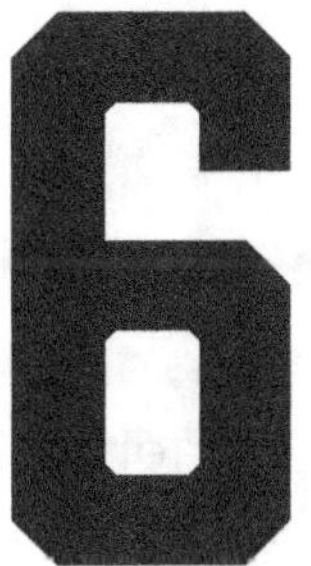

TOURNIQUET

In the context of Tactical Medicine, the use of a tourniquet has proven effective in stopping bleeding. A distinction is made between two different phases. The best known is that of an initial application to stop severe, life-threatening bleeding on the extremities immediately and efficiently. The tourniquet is applied as high (proximal) as possible and as tight as necessary. "High and tight" is the key phrase here. The tourniquet is also applied above the clothing, but only when the pockets are empty. It is important to secure the tourniquet against unintentional or deliberate loosening and to record the application time. Further possible errors are listed below.

The second option for applying a tourniquet is the last resort in case all the alternatives for stopping bleeding (see 6.2 and 6.3) have not produced the desired result.

There are now well over a dozen tourniquets on the market, and it is difficult to find the right one. As part of the TCCC Guidelines, recommendations are published by coTCCC to provide guidance. Ultimately, the choice of an individual tourniquet is a personal decision. One must be able to work with it themselves; above all, both variants, application to oneself and to others, should be feasible.

TEN TOURNIQUET APPLICATION MISTAKES

1. **TOO LATE:**
   The rescuer hesitates too long.

2. **LAX SECURING:**
   This prevents efficient hemostasis.

3. **LACK OF PRE-TENSIONING:**
   This causes technical problems.

4. **FAILURE TO SECURE THE EXCESS LENGTHS:**
   Resulting in unintentional opening.

5. **NO SECURING OF THE TIMING BAND.**

6. **NO RECORDING OF THE APPLICATION TIME.**

7. **NO CLEARING OF THE LEG POCKETS:**
   Resulting in incorrect application.

8. **APPLICATION POINT TOO LOW, RESULTING IN A LACK OF COMPRESSION.**

9. **USE OF IMPROVISED AND DEFECTIVE TOURNIQUETS, SUCH AS PLAGIARIZED PRODUCTS.**

10. **POSITIONING OF THE TOGGLE IN THE GROIN, UNABLE TO ROTATE IT.**

THE TOURNIQUET

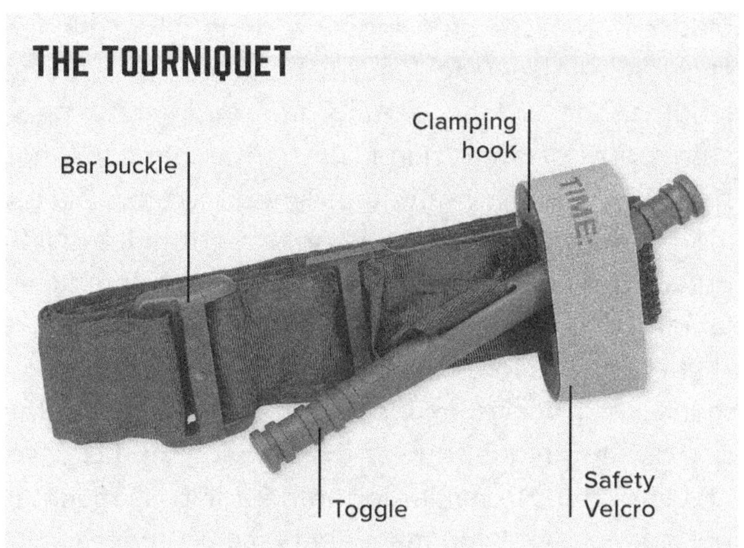

PRESSURE DRESSINGS AND JUNCTIONAL BLEEDING

Only very few bleeding wounds actually require the permanent application of a tourniquet. In most cases, hemostasis can be achieved with a well-applied pressure dressing. Even if the doctrine that a tourniquet should only be removed by a doctor or medical professional is stubbornly maintained in military and police training, converting, i.e. replacing a tourniquet with a pressure wound dressing, should be practiced. The so-called ischemic pain, i.e. the pain caused by the tourniquet itself, is, in some cases, unbearable for the person affected after just a few minutes. Injured people, therefore, often try to open a tourniquet themselves. For this reason alone, the possibility of replacing it should be known.

Modern pressure dressings are generally designed similarly: an elastic gauze bandage of varying lengths, one or more wound dressings, and a pressure body of some kind. Once the bandage has been unwound, it can be easily secured (usually using a hook). It is easy to use on the extremities without much practice. It is more difficult in the so-called junctional areas of the neck, armpit, and groin.

In some cases, massive bleeding can occur at these sites due to injuries, which do not allow the use of a tourniquet due to the location. In this case, it is important to minimize the bleeding as much as possible by applying manual pressure **(finger in the wound or fist on the feeding artery).** This must always be practiced. The pressure bandage that is then applied must also be taught professionally and practiced repeatedly. It is all too easy for user errors to creep in here, which can lead to fatal results in a real emergency situation. **Hemostyptic** agents are often included in this type of care.

HEMOSTYPTICS

One achievement of modern times is the invention and further development of so-called hemostyptic dressings. There are currently two market-dominating types of active ingredients, which are distributed and used in a somewhat wider range of applications due to different carrier systems and application variants. Originally sprinkled into the wound as granules, with the side effect of increased thermal reaction, they are now available for vaporization or drenching absorbent gauze or compresses without negative side effects.

Whether Chitosan or Kaolin products, both materials belong to the group of hemostyptic agents, are introduced into deep wound cavities by means of so-called wound packs and support the effect of natural blood clotting under pressure. The effects of improved and accelerated blood coagulation differ as follows:

Type	Mechanism	Additional info
Chitosan	Combination of positively and negatively charged components	Works even in blood with a low coagulation factor
Kaolin	Support of coagulation factors through natural minerals	Body-warm blood is necessary

STOPPING BLEEDING: APPLYING THE TOURNIQUET CORRECTLY

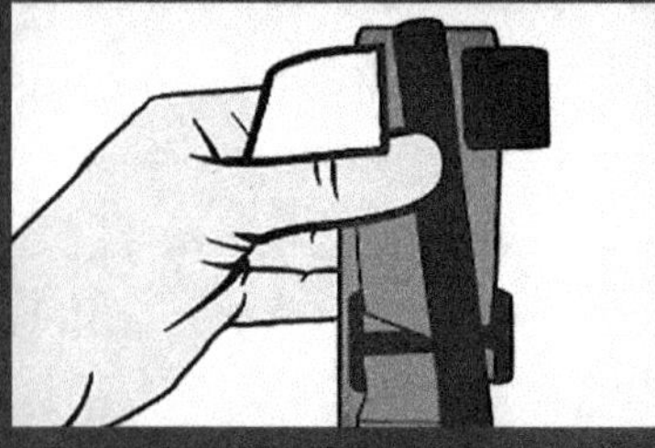

Remove the tourniquet from the IFAK or the carrying bag. We show a CAT in action.

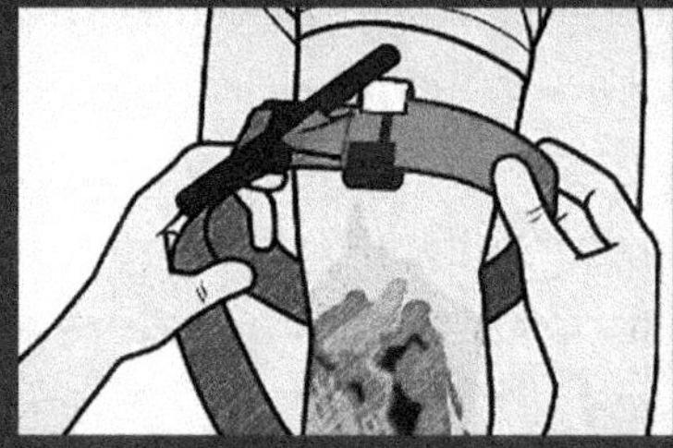

Pass the injured arm or leg through the loop of the Velcro strap.

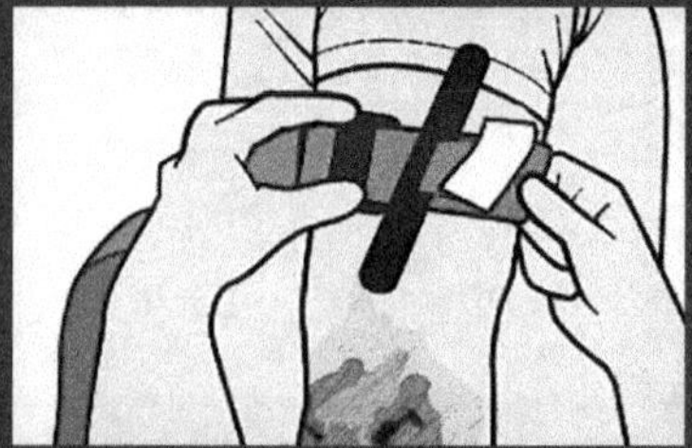

Arms or legs are tied off as high as possible so that nothing is overlooked.

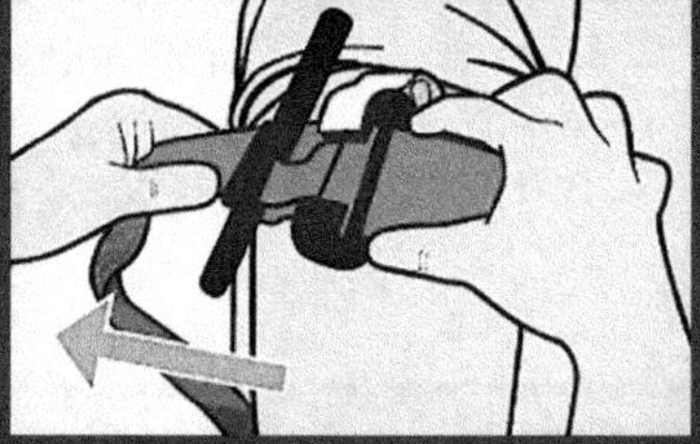

Pull the free end of the tourniquet strap as tightly as possible around the limb.

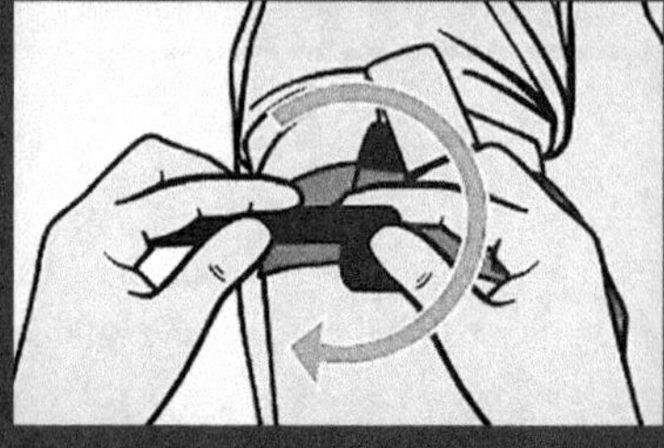

Turn the toggle until the strap is fully tightened to stop the bleeding.

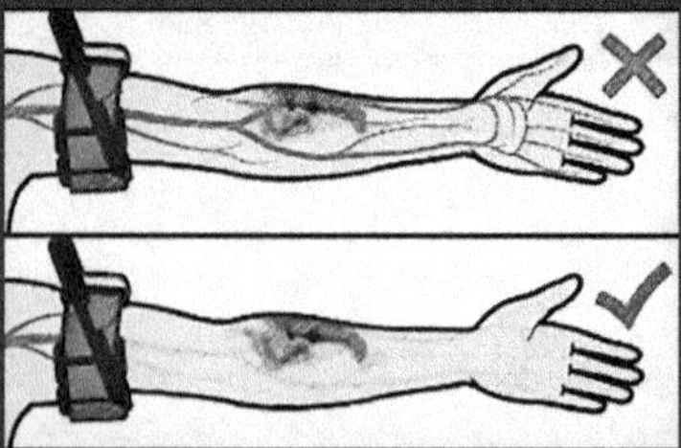

If the tourniquet is not properly tightened, the bleeding will not stop. Very tight means very safe.

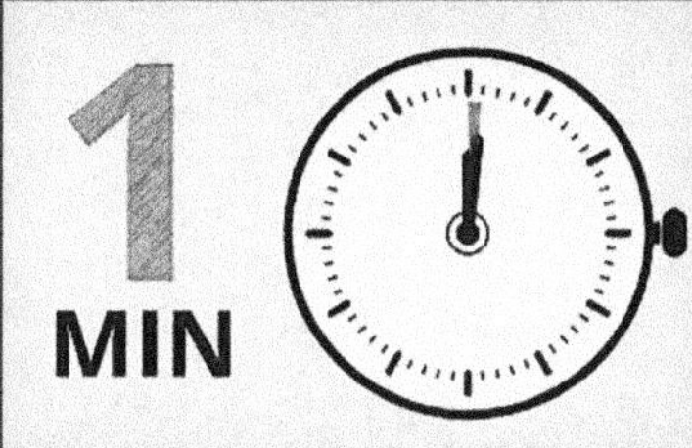

If applied correctly, the tourniquet will stop the bleeding within one minute.

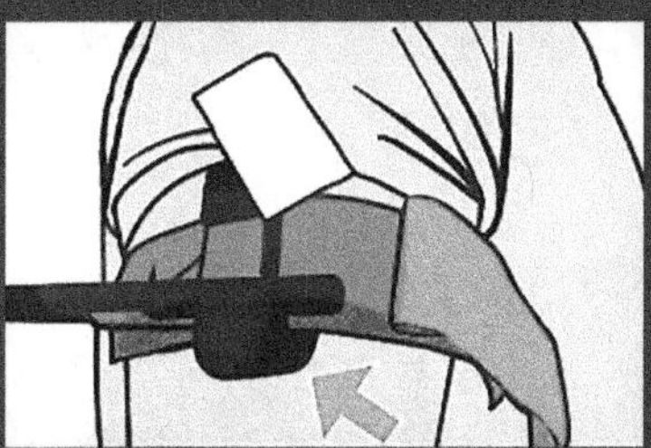

The toggle must be secured to the safety hook in order to remain securely tightened.

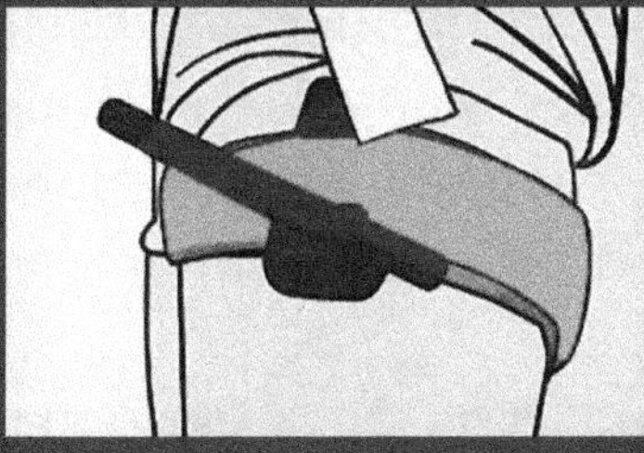

The Velcro strap of the tourniquet runs through the securing hook and past the toggle.

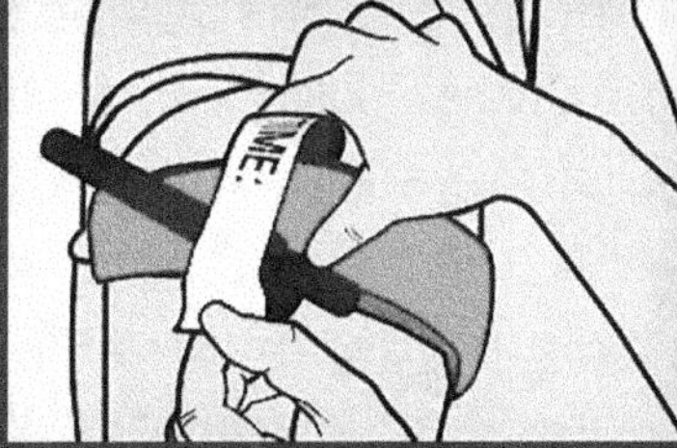

The toggle and Velcro strap of the tourniquet are then secured with the safety Velcro.

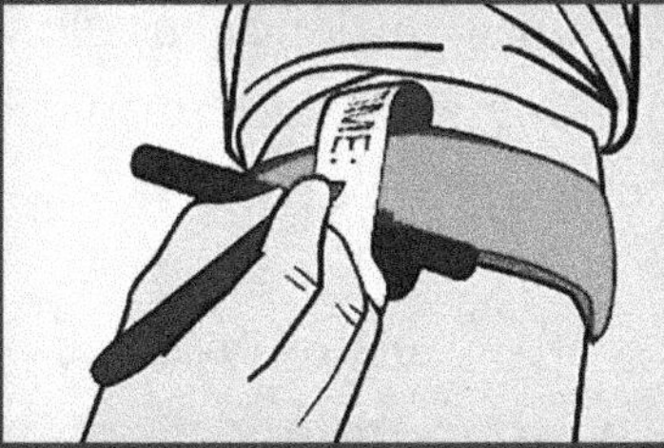

The time of application is noted both on the safety strap and the casualty card.

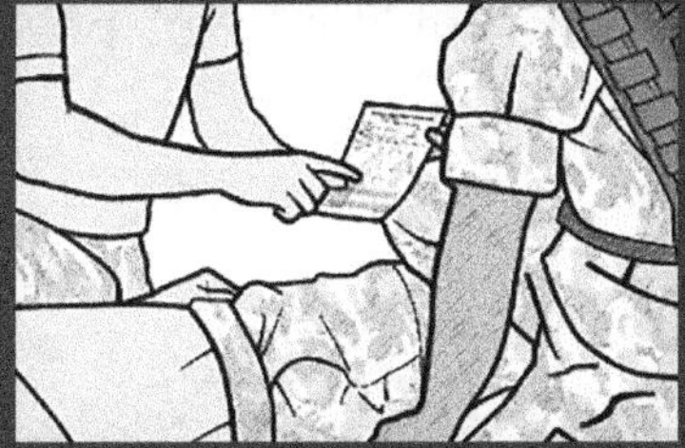

Upon delivery, explain to the medical staff what is known about the injuries.

AIRWAY MANAGEMENT 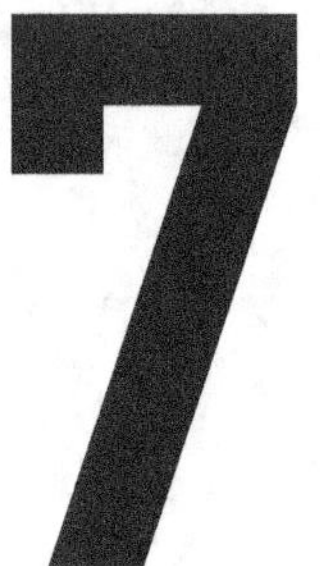

NPA / OPA

After life-threatening bleeding, opening the airway or keeping it open is the second-most important task in Tactical Medicine. There are various options for escalation. In principle, basic measures such as the Heimlich maneuver or coma position are used in TCCC treatment as well. However, the major challenge is often evacuation and securing the measures taken.

The application of a **Wendl tube** (NPA, Nasopharyngeal Airways) is already considered under the letter **A (Airways)** for unconscious or severely disoriented patients. This is intended to keep the airways open, but does not provide any protection against aspiration. This invasive application also requires practice and is frequently characterized by failure, especially for first-aiders.

The **Guedel tube** (OPA, Oropharyngeal Airways), which is frequently used in emergency medical services and clinical settings, plays a subordinate role in Tactical Medicine. Although it is typically easier to use and does not require as much training, its fixation is questionable and inefficient, especially during an evacuation. In addition, the OPA does not provide aspiration protection either.

I-GEL TUBES OR MASKS

The TCCC guidelines also include recommendations for the use of so-called **i-gel products,** such as **i-gel masks** and **i-gel tubes**. These products can be found in the extended spectrum, especially at a higher specialist level, where their use makes sense. At the lowest level of TCCC/TECC qualification, it is rather unusual to carry these airway materials, as their use is not part of the corresponding basic training.

EMERGENCY CRICOTHYROTOMY

Injury patterns such as severe mid-face trauma are quite common in the Tactical Medicine spectrum compared to standard civilian rescue services. Massive trauma to the head, but also strong pressures caused by explosions (blast), very often cause the upper airways to fail due to swelling or complete deformation. In such a situation, the creation of a so-called surgical airway access is a necessity. Emergency cricothyrotomy ("cricing") is therefore also trained at the extended user level of TCCC. This is necessary because, due to tactical circumstances, specialist medical personnel are only deployed at a later stage.

This procedure must be practiced regularly, as it certainly cannot be described as a simple first-aid measure. Although there are industrially manufactured "cric sets" that significantly minimize the error rate when performing the procedure, the basic measures for securing the airway should not be ignored either.

SUMMARY:

After stopping the bleeding, the most important task of a first-aider is to clear the airway or keep it clear. In addition to the basic measures of general first aid, there are also extended options available with or without the use of materials. It is imperative that this intervention be properly trained and regularly practiced in order to be successful in an emergency.

HEAT PRESERVATION

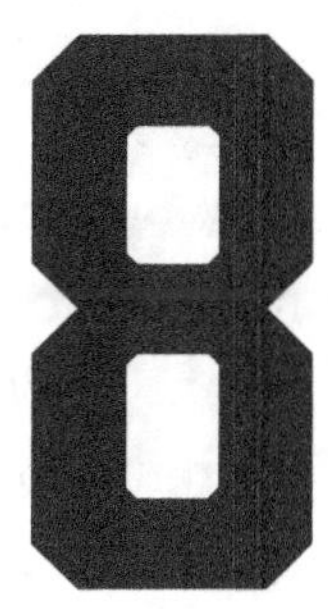

THE PROBLEM OF HYPOTHERMIA IS AN EXTREMELY IMPORTANT TOPIC IN TACTICAL MEDICINE.

Due to the experience gained in dealing with cooled or hypothermic casualties, a clear focus is placed on this. This certainly distinguishes Tactical Medicine from the regular rescue service, which, with pre-warmed rescue equipment and usually short transport times, is unlikely to enter the danger zone of hypothermia. This makes it all the more essential to raise awareness and provide materials for hypothermia prophylaxis and heat therapy. Such awareness is frequently not present among helpers, as they themselves sweat heavily under the strain of providing care and their own equipment, and therefore hardly realize that the wounded person is cooling down. Ambient temperatures, such as those prevailing in Africa or Afghanistan, also lead to the misconception that the patient must be warm.

However, even if the ground is dry, it is generally much cooler than the human body, which leads to a latent flow of body heat downward. In this way, the human body loses a great deal of heat and energy. Loosely covering the body with a rescue blanket can therefore only be regarded as suboptimal. When attempting to keep the patient warm, it is always important to think outside the box and include any aids from the surrounding area. Euro pallets, cardboard boxes, or whatever is available to the rescuer serves its purpose in preventing cooling. Ultimately, this cooling leads to the injured person's blood clotting steadily deteriorating. The rule of thumb here is that for every degree of body temperature, ten percent of the body's own blood coagulation is lost. So what good is the best bandage if life-threatening bleeding starts again due to inadequate heat retention?

RESCUE BLANKET

The rescue blanket, also known as a NASA blanket, is a universal tool. Originally developed for space travel, as the name suggests, it was first used as a warming blanket during the New York Marathon in the 1970s. We are all familiar with this function from first-aid kits alone. However, reducing this blanket to this function alone does not do it justice. Joint projects with the Tyrol Mountain Rescue Service have identified up to eight other "off-label" functions for which this rescue blanket can be used. Here we are focusing on heat retention. Unfortunately, it is usually used incorrectly for this purpose.

Placing the rescue blanket over an injured person and simply covering them with it is at best sufficient, but the result is rather inadequate. The **<u>diaper principle</u>,"** i.e., pulling the blanket through between two layers of clothing and then bringing it together by pulling it through between the legs up to the abdomen, describes this principle quite well. The rescue blanket covers the entire back, the genital area, the front of the body, and, if necessary, the head when formed into a hood. In total, this type of heat retention covers around 60 to 70 percent of the body surface. As a positive side effect, a rescue blanket placed in this way will remain in place even when moving during an evacuation or patient transport and will also remain stable in strong winds, such as a helicopter's downwash.

The frequently asked question of which side should point towards the patient and which away from the patient is pretty irrelevant, as there are hardly any serious differences. According to the manufacturer, silver should point towards the patient.

BLIZZARD BLANKET

The blizzard blanket is basically a further development of the rescue blanket described above. However, this blizzard blanket is much more stable, and its overall surface structure is significantly larger due to the honeycomb structure. The advantage of this is that air warmed by the human body has more volume and can provide a correspondingly higher heat output. Just imagine the grooved structure of sheet metal and compare it with smooth surfaces. The principle is the same. The disadvantages of the blizzard blanket are its large pack size and its higher weight compared to the aforementioned rescue blanket. However, this should not be an obstacle on a vehicle. The blizzard blanket is also available as a hood or poncho.

APLS TRANSPORT BAG

The APLS (Absorbent Patient Litter System), available in winter and summer versions, is a good way of combining patient transportation and heat retention. The winter version is more heavily padded, and the bag can also be closed with a zipper. The transport handles are also much more sturdily sewn. The summer version can be closed with Velcro strips and has no padding. Due to these features, however, it is also significantly smaller and lighter in its packaging.

Both APLS variants allow a patient to be packed and transported while being protected from the weather. The APLS bag is certainly a significant improvement compared to conventional transportation or rescue cloths, if only because of the additional thermal protection.

READY HEAT BLANKET

All the products mentioned so far make it possible to preserve the residual heat of the human body. They are not an active way of warming the body. The Ready Heat Blanket, in its various sizes, can generate exactly this: an active warming of the human body by means of chemical reactions in the pads of the blanket. Basically, this is what we know from the chemical heat bags of hand warmers. The reaction with air leads to the production of heat. Up to a maximum of 45 degrees of heat can actively warm a chilled patient. In combination with an APLS bag or a blizzard blanket, this is a very good way of combating cooling even in cold temperatures. The difficulty is the use of Ready Heat at altitudes above 2500 meters above sea level, as the oxygen content decreases there. At high altitudes, Ready Heat therefore loses some of its heat output.

SUMMARY:

The deterioration of patients' general condition after trauma due to loss of body heat (loss of blood as a heat regulator) or insufficient protection against ambient cold or wetness is called hypothermia. Actively counteracting this hypothermia, if possible, or at least preventing its progression, is one of the most important tasks in first aid. This is why maintaining warmth is the third-most significant measure after stopping bleeding and securing the airway.

INFUSION LINES

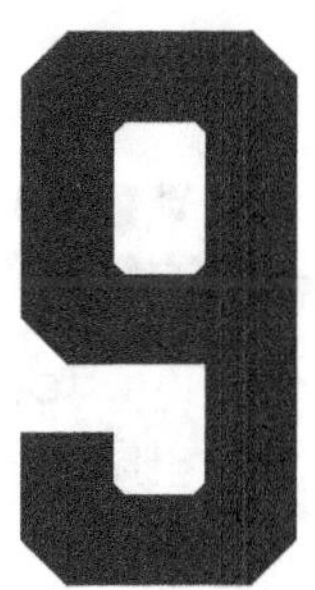

ONE OF THE POSSIBLE FORMS OF THERAPY FOR TREATING THE WOUNDED IN TACTICAL MEDICINE IS THE CREATION OF LINES.

Infusion fluids and medication can be administered via these lines. The basic rule in Tactical Medicine is that every patient gets a line, but not everyone gets fluids. Opinions are certainly divided on this, but if you consider the frequently prolonged evacuation times and possible complications, this statement is perhaps self-explanatory.

There are basically two different approaches to creating access for the application of medical compounds. Which one you personally favor depends on many aspects: the Tactical Medical situation, material resources, protocols of your own organization, the medical condition of the patient himself, and your own ability to carry out the procedure.

INTRAVENOUS

Intravenous (IV) lines should always be the standard. Whether in clinical or preclinical settings, IV lines are normally used everywhere. The choice of a puncture site and the size of the **intravenous venous catheter** may differ. The size and thus the **flow rate** (volume size) are specified in **gauge** (G). The following is an overview of common sizes:

Color	Length in mm	Size in gauge	Flow rate in ml/min
YELLOW	19	24	22
BLUE	25	22	36
PINK	33	20	61
GREEN	45	18	96
WHITE	45	17	128
GREY	50	16	196
ORANGE	50	14	343

There are also winged infusion sets ("Butterflies"), which are mostly used in pediatric medicine and are of secondary importance due to their low flow rate. Nevertheless, it is good to have such Butterflies with you, as it is easier to puncture veins with their short and fine needles than with the larger cannulas mentioned above.

As already mentioned, creating an IV line does not necessarily mean that fluids need to be infused. In many cases, a mandrin is inserted into the cannula to keep the access open, i.e., to protect it from being blocked by blood clots. If the vascular levels of the wounded person change in the further course of events so that fluids or medication need to be administered, the line is available and can usually be cleared again by simple flushing with saline solution.

INTRAOSSEOUS

Intraosseous (IO) lines are more common in Tactical Medicine than in standard medical services. The reasons for this are complex. On the one hand, it is often easier for untrained first-aiders to handle the applicator to insert a steel mandrin into a bone than to perform the more delicate task of tapping a vein that may have already collapsed due to blood loss. In addition, systems for creating an IO line are now very user-friendly.

However, there is a rule of thumb to follow:

2:2
TWO UNSUCCESSFUL ATTEMPTS TO FIND AN INTRAVENOUS LINE, OR TWO MINUTES OF UNSUCCESSFULLY SEARCHING A VEIN FOR TAPPING.

Both result in too much time elapsing before the wounded person receives fluids.

As with IV access materials, there are different materials for IO access. The two most commonly used are the **EZ IO,** an applicator very similar to a small hand drill, and the **FAST-1** system, a pressure plunger with a retaining ring.

ERRORS WHEN PUNCTURING VEINS:

▶ missing tourniquet;
▶ inadequate disinfection of the puncture site;
▶ poor preparation of the gear, including plaster strips;
▶ too late application, collapsed veins;
▶ incorrect choice of venous cannulas (too large, too small);
▶ incorrect or inappropriate puncture site;
▶ excessive tightening of the skin, resulting in flattening of the vein;
▶ poor lighting and visibility;

- puncture angle too steep or too shallow (ideal: 30°);
- steel cannula is withdrawn too late or too early;
- unsure, slow advancement of the plastic cannula;
- poor and improper fixation of the venous cannula.

ERRORS WHEN PUNCTURING BONE MARROW:

- wrong puncture site;
- inadequate disinfection;
- poor preparation of the gear;
- incorrect puncture angle (90° to the body surface);
- too weak, timid trigger pressure during puncture;
- lack of aspiration after puncture;
- lack of irrigation after puncture;
- missing three-way stopcock;
- incorrect position of the three-way stopcock;
- incorrect line fixation.

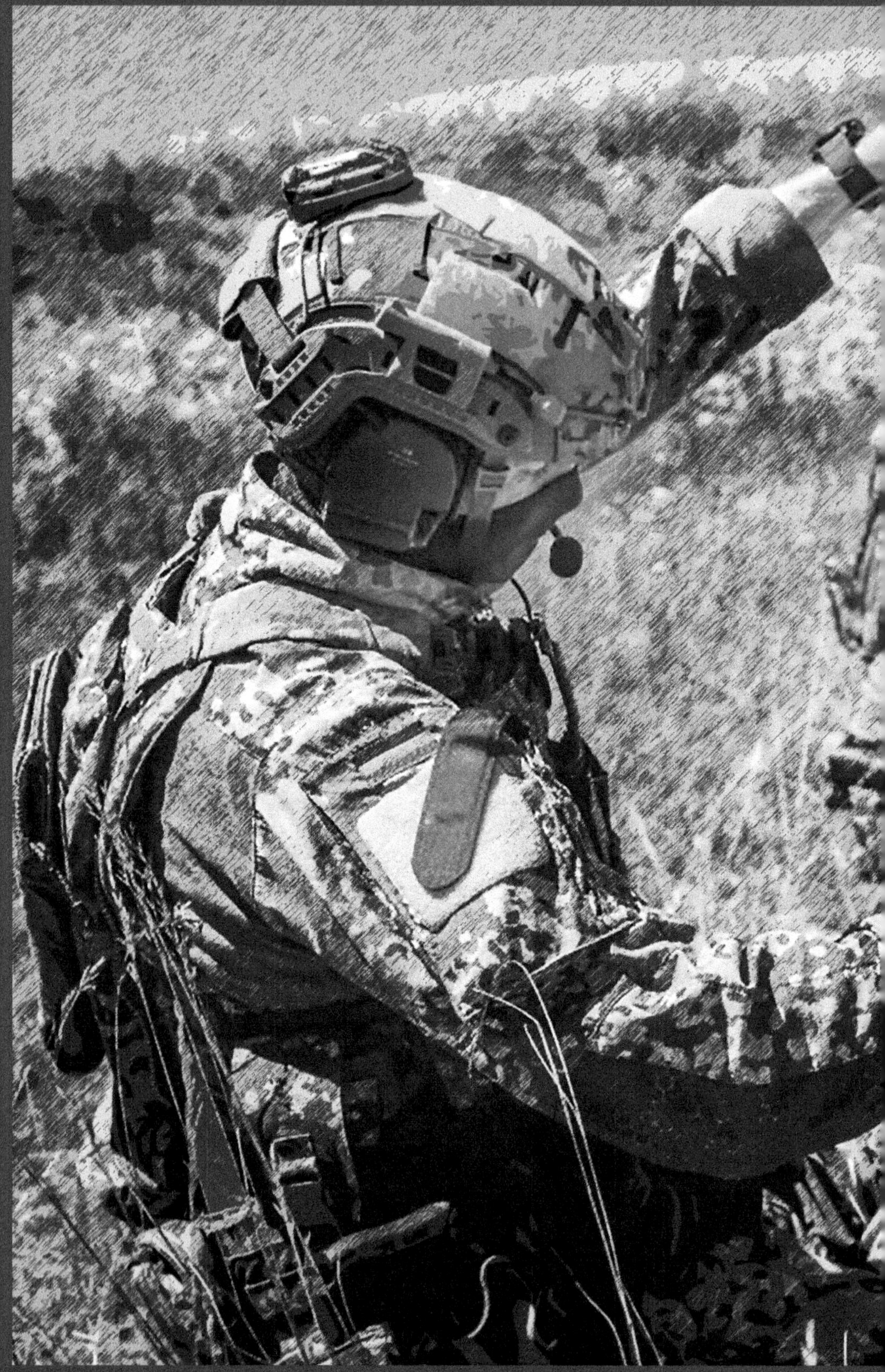

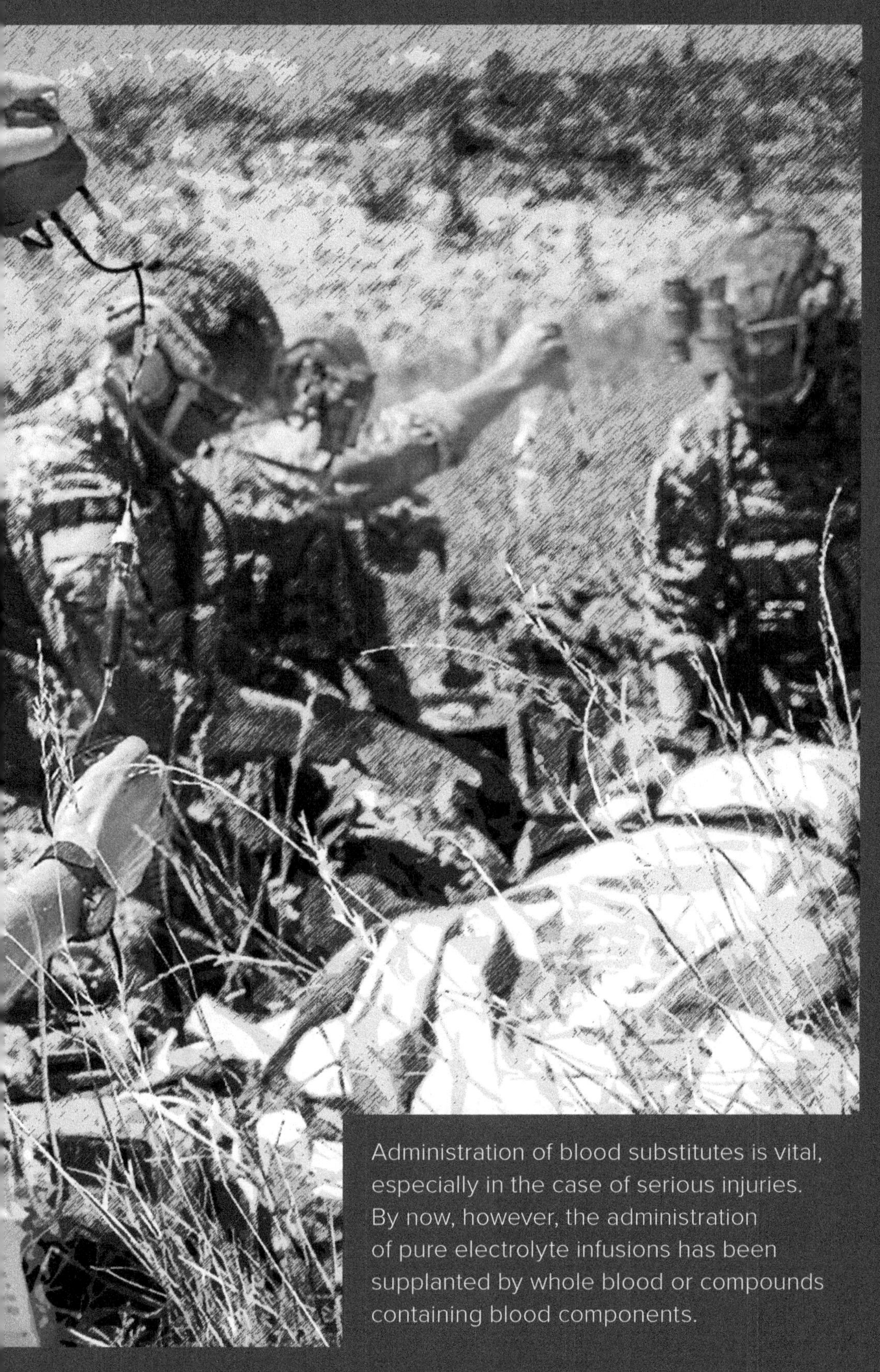

Administration of blood substitutes is vital, especially in the case of serious injuries. By now, however, the administration of pure electrolyte infusions has been supplanted by whole blood or compounds containing blood components.

SUMMARY:

Intravenous or intraosseous lines are invasive measures and require legal clearance, especially for nonmedical personnel. In most cases, the respective protocols of the organizations regulate such clearance. In addition, these measures must be practiced regularly. Various sources speak of a considerable number of errors in the preclinical application of intraosseous lines, as several physical steps are necessary. One of those intermediate steps is often executed incorrectly or simply forgotten, e.g., flushing after the tap to create space in the bone marrow for the infusion fluid itself. These steps are best practiced under more stressful conditions than in the classroom!

FRACTURE SPLINTING 10

NOT EXACTLY AT THE TOP OF THE LIST, THE TREATMENT OF FRACTURES IS OFTEN PUSHED FAR BACK IN THE SEQUENCE OF INDIVIDUAL TREATMENT STEPS.

Fractures are regularly very difficult to reliably diagnose at the prehospital stage, making it very complex for the rescuer to decide what to do first. Concentrating on stopping bleeding, airway management, and maintaining warmth, a rescuer very quickly reaches his limits when confronted with fractures, as the patient himself shows him the limits of what he can do due to the pain. Irritated by this and hindered in his or her scheme, the caregiver typically tries to treat fractures somehow, oftentimes ineffectively. Nevertheless, the treatment of fractures is fundamentally important, as improperly handled fractures can lead to secondary injuries, sometimes with massive to life-threatening bleeding, or other serious accompanying problems, such as fat embolisms. As we do not have X-ray vision, every injured person with indications of a safe but also unsafe fracture must first be treated as an injured person with a fracture.

SAFE AND UNSAFE FRACTURE SIGNS:

SAFE

- ▶ open perforation of the skin, visible fracture ends
- ▶ abnormal position of the limb
- ▶ abnormal mobility of the limb

UNSAFE

- ▶ pain
- ▶ swelling
- ▶ bruises (hematoma)
- ▶ hampered movement

Possible blood loss due to fractures:

Forearm	500 ml
Upper arm	800 ml
Lower leg	800 ml
Thigh	2000 ml
Pelvis	5000 ml

PREFAB SPLINTS

Tactical Medical personnel should ideally have the appropriate professional equipment at their disposal. Conventional splint procedures have been common materials for treating most fractures for many years. It is usually possible to immobilize the two joints adjacent to the fracture site. Fixation using triangular cloth ties or other tools has proven effective for this purpose. Sensitive areas of the body are often padded using the soft padding material of the splint itself. This splint material is flexible and only becomes stable when folded several times. It is available rolled or folded. The water-repellent surface material also makes it reusable. Due to their light weight, splints of this type can also be stowed in any smaller medic pack or rucksack system. Some of them come with printed instructions on how to use them in different ways.

IMPROVISED SPLINTS

Improper handling of fractures can cause pain, exacerbate a possible shock, or cause additional internal bleeding by injuring blood vessels running parallel to the fracture ends. These reasons speak in favor of splinting or at least immobilizing every fracture, even if one is only suspected. There are various materials available for this purpose, both from everyday life and from nature. The "off-label" use of a wide variety of items as fracture splints should also be part of extended paramedic training. From pieces of clothing, magazines, or rucksacks to boards or branches, there are a lot of items with the potential for splinting. Even or especially when using improvised materials, care must be taken to ensure that sensitive contact points, such as joints, are properly padded. Nerve damage can be triggered very quickly by punctual pressure. Care should also be taken in advance to avoid pointed or sharp objects. Remember as well that the healthy second leg can be used for splinting!

THE MOST COMMON ERRORS IN SPLINTING FRACTURES:

1. INCORRECT, INAPPROPRIATE SPLINTING MATERIAL;

2. INCORRECT REPOSITIONING OF THE TWO ADJACENT JOINTS;

3. LOOSE SPLINTING;

4. SPLINTING IN AN ABNORMAL POSITION;

5. UNCOVERED, OPEN FRACTURE ENDS;

6. FAILURE TO CONTROL BLOOD CIRCULATION, MOTOR FUNCTION, AND SENSITIVITY;

7. FAILURE TO PAD JOINTS;

8. FIXATION KNOTS PLACED ON JOINTS;

9. LACK OF TRACTION DURING FIXATION AFTER REPOSITIONING;

10. LACK OF COMMUNICATION WITH THE INJURED PERSON.

The repositioning of a fracture is an exceptional situation in the standard pre-hospital rescue service. In the field of Tactical Medicine, this complex measure occurs more frequently. The need to carry out sometimes complex evacuations over long distances can only be performed with extremities in a normal position. The time factor also plays a role in the need to ensure blood circulation and sensitivity within a broken limb. It is important to learn this measure professionally in advance and to approach the problem with the will to carry it out to the end. Once the initially painful traction has been applied to a fractured limb, the fracture ends must remain in traction and thus be fixed.

Another special feature is the splinting or immobilization of a possible pelvic fracture. Patients with such a life-threatening fracture reach the emergency room of a hospital with a very high error rate. This means that many indications of such an injury are not recognized by first-aiders. Based on this, first responders in Tactical Medicine receive significantly more training in recognizing and treating such injuries. The potential for internal bleeding resulting from pelvic fractures is excessively high.

A FEW SIGNS OF PELVIC FRACTURES:

- ▶ **kinematics;**
- ▶ **contusion marks (hematomas in the pelvic area);**
- ▶ **clear misalignment of the iliac crest (hip bone);**
- ▶ **pain in the pelvic area;**
- ▶ **high amputation (above the ankle joint);**
- ▶ **gunshot or splinter injuries in the pelvic area, but also in the abdomen.**

The mere indication of one of these possible signs is sufficient reason to immobilize the pelvis. Professional aids, such as pelvic slings from various suppliers, but also the improvised variant using a rescue blanket, are available for this purpose. The use of such aids must be practiced, and, if possible, such treatment should be carried out by two helpers.

SUMMARY:
Fractures are not only painful conditions; they can also very quickly lead to life-threatening situations and exacerbate shock. Splinting fractures requires technical skill and anatomical background knowledge. These are things that can be learned and mastered through regular practice. Unfortunately, however, very few first-aiders are able to splint fractures sufficiently pre-hospital.

RESCUE AND EVACUATION 11

"RESCUE AND EVACUATION" IS A VERY BROAD COLLECTIVE TERM FOR VARIOUS ACTIVITIES IN TACTICAL MEDICINE.

It can describe rescue operations and transportation options in the Care Under Fire phase, but also the handover of an injured person in the final phase, Tactical Evacuation Care. For this reason, the respective terms are described in more detail in the following subsections.

TRANSPORT HOLDS

Moving casualties from one point to another in any way is often a challenge for everyone involved. Tactical conditions, such as direct or indirect fire, terrain profiles, type of injury, cooperation of the patient, and the number and physical robustness of the helpers, are just some key aspects that limit the choice of procedure for transporting casualties.

As they are typically very physically demanding, such transport maneuvers are rarely practiced during training. In principle, a clear distinction must be made as to which transport hold should be used in which phase. For the benefit of all, a clear decision must be made here, depending on the situation. If the rescuer and patient are in an acutely dangerous situation, a further distinction must be made. Quick exit with the use of simple maneuvers that are usually not very gentle on the patient (crash rescue), or low/high crawl? This clearly shows how much influence the threat situation has on the procedure itself. While the **Fireman's Carry** (the casualty is thrown over the shoulder of the rescuer) and the **Rautek Hold** are the best-known transport holds in crash rescues, the crawling approach, which is much more laborious to execute, offers a number of variants. Resting on the thigh, grabbing down the back of the neck, or dragging at the equipment are just three of the many more **drag tricks** in low/high crawl. As already mentioned, this is nothing that would be practiced with pleasure. The use of webbing loops, tents, straps, or harnesses can also be useful here. It simply needs to be practiced.

It goes without saying that transportation is easier and faster for two people. If a third helper is added, the wounded can almost be evacuated on the move: The patient is placed on the two front carriers, the legs are placed on the third man's shoulders, and off you go. Two helpers can carry a wounded man sitting upright and grabbing the shoulders of the rescuers easily and fast. This obviously assumes that the injured person is at least cooperative.

MEANS OF TRANSPORTATION

There seem to be hardly any limits to the choice of aids for transporting injured persons. Industrially manufactured or improvised: Whatever is available should be used in an emergency. So think and practice unconventionally during training. Tried-and-tested systems—in many wars—are the classic **stretchers.** Even though they have certainly changed in terms of stability and weight in recent years, their basic design and application remain largely unchanged. At least two, more likely four carriers—four men, four handles, and off you go. It is important that the injured person is able to look in the direction of travel. Also, do not walk in lockstep if possible. It is also essential that one person give the command when lifting and setting down. Otherwise, it will be uncomfortable for the person lying on the stretcher. Whenever possible, the injured person should be secured to the stretcher using restraining straps. Unfortunately, despite the fact that such stretchers have been in use for so long, it has not yet been possible to establish a standardized measure. As a result, it is often necessary to reposition injured persons, as the stretcher in question is not compatible with the rescue vehicle's stretcher carriage.

In addition to stretchers, there are also numerous **slings.** Those are also very different. Designed for different patient weights, from light and flexible in pack size to rigid and heavy, everything is available. The choice of sling is therefore a very individual one. Simply try out different systems and then decide. Basically, the benefits of a transport sling should also be weighed against the size of the equipment. It is possible to improvise with the transport sling as well. A **makeshift stretcher** using **field jackets,** blankets, and sturdy carrying poles is not the worst option. Such makeshift stretchers are also well suited for transporting material.

One of the lightest transport options, which is usually also available for units operating with limited additional equipment, is working with webbing loops or ropes. The term **"Hasty Harness"** is used to describe a number of procedures for transporting casualties with the aid of such leashes and ropes. This is a practice-intensive procedure that, if not repeated regularly, is more likely to cause confusion than provide relief.

Another collective term for different types of stretchers is the "roll-up" stretcher. As the name suggests, this is a stretcher that is transported rolled up in the transport rucksack, unrolled after removal, and then stabilized by means of cross braces. Simpler versions do not include cross stabilizers and are therefore only used to transport casualties quickly and swiftly, supported by holding loops for the rescuers. The more stable versions may even have a winch connection and are good rescue equipment for use in difficult terrain. The same applies here as with the slings: The overall scope of the operational equipment also determines the selection of the **"roll-up" carrying system.**

SUMMARY:
There are many options for transporting casualties. The tactical deployment and the resulting limiting factors regarding weight and volume determine their selection. As is so often the case in Tactical Medicine, off-label use and improvised procedures are important additions that can ultimately lead to the successful transportation of an injured person.

REPORTING SCHEMES

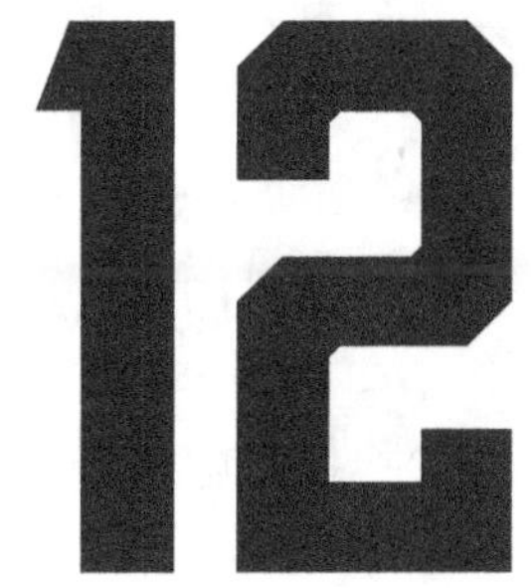

THE 9 LINE MEDEVAC REQUEST IS A TERM THAT HAS BEEN FREQUENTLY USED IN RECENT YEARS IN CONNECTION WITH THE DEPLOYMENT OF RESCUE HELICOPTERS.

Mistakenly, a direct connection between 9 Line and helicopter deployment has crept in as a fixed value. In principle, 9 Line does not decide on the means of rescue but serves as the basis for transmitting a radio message. Such radio messages were originally sent in accordance with NATO Standard Operating Procedure using the METHANE (7 Line) scheme. METHANE has fallen somewhat into the background due to its use in the context of ISAF (International

Security Assistance Force) and RS (Resolute Support) in Afghanistan and the low level of use there. Nevertheless, both are still common radio schemes in NATO manuals, e.g., according to NATO Standard ATP 3.3.2.1.

METHANE

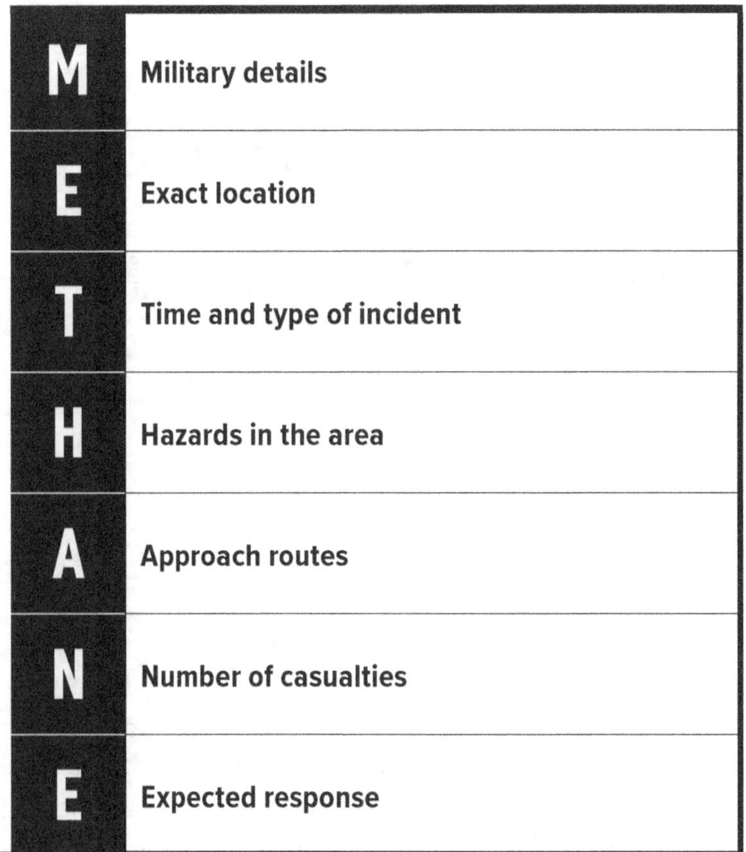

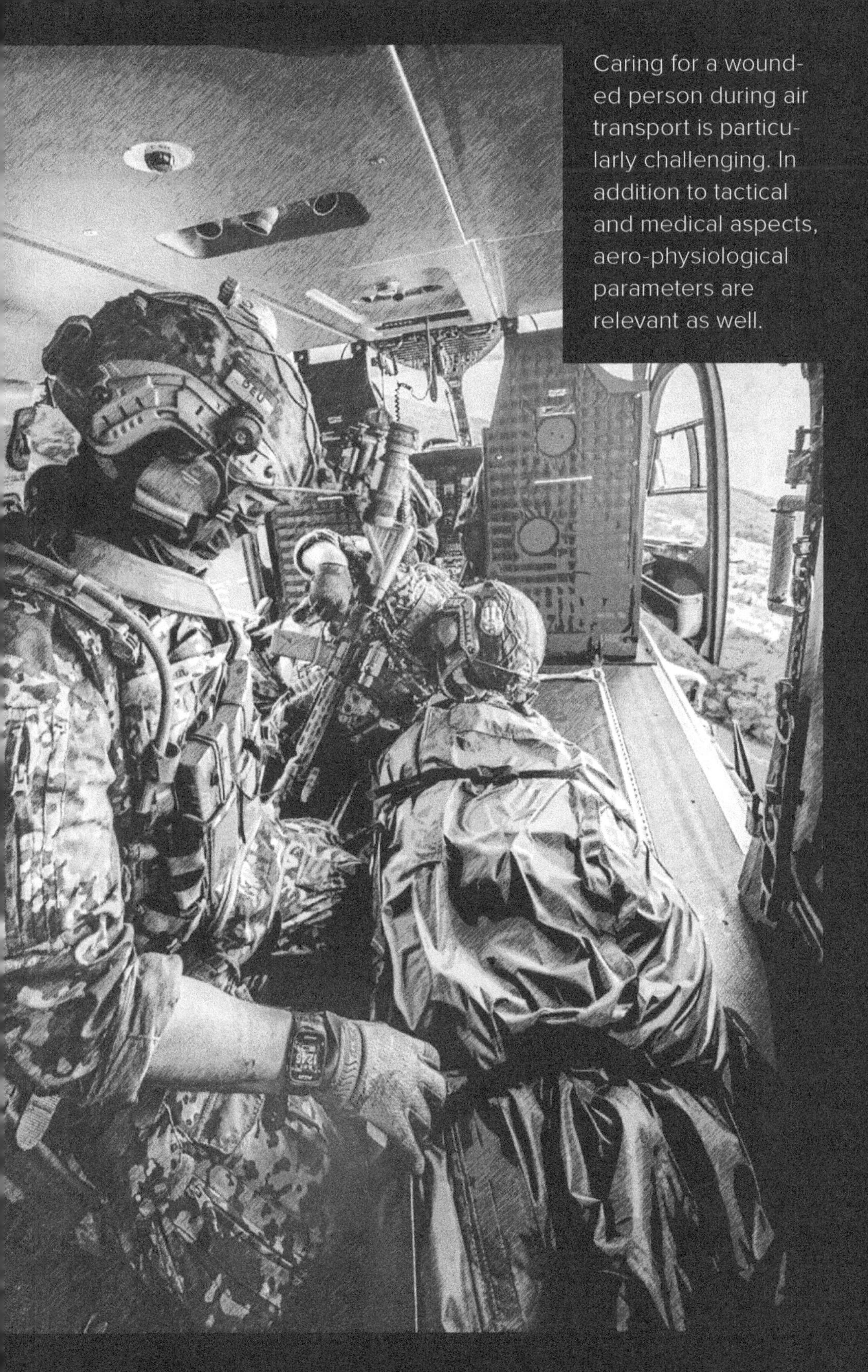

Caring for a wound-
ed person during air
transport is particu-
larly challenging. In
addition to tactical
and medical aspects,
aero-physiological
parameters are
relevant as well.

9 LINE

Line 1	**Location of pickup site**
Line 2	**Radio call sign and frequency**
Line 3	**No. of patients by urgency** **A** Urgent **B** Priority **C** Routine
Line 4	**Special equipment required** **A** NONE **B** Hoist **C** Extraction equipment **D** Ventilation
Line 5	**No. of patients by type** **A** Litter **B** Ambulatory

Line 6	**Security at pickup site** (in peace: no. and type of wounds)
Line 7	**Method of marking pickup site** **A** Panels **B** Pyrotechnics **C** Smoke **D** None **E** Other
Line 8	**Patient Nationality** **A** U.S. military **B** U.S. civilian **C** Non-U.S. military **D** Non-U.S. civilian **E** EPW
Line 9	**CBRNe threat** (in peace: terrain description)

The use of these two radio templates has made a significant contribution to minimizing error rates and range interference caused by language barriers. Both radio stations are provided with the respective scheme, which enables the respective line to be filled in easily without repeating the question. Electronic data transfer makes filling in the pre-prepared data forms much faster and more efficient. Tactical leaders in particular, who are involved in an incident with casualties, have little time and capacity for complex radio procedures. Lines 3 and 4 (9 Line) are provided by medical personnel; the rest is their business. The categorization of the wounded according to A, B, and C should be left to professionally trained personnel. The assignment of categories makes sense, especially with limited high-value resources, in order to avoid tying up high-value rescue forces in minor cases.

CAT A	**Urgent** (Evacuation required within two hours)
CAT B	**Priority** (Evacuation required within four hours)
CAT C	**Routine** (Evacuation required within 24 hours)

Afghanistan's experiences have led to the recommendation that line 7 should only be sketchy, e.g., C for SMOKE, and the color of the smoke used should then be named as a kind of confirmation on site. Radio transmissions were often intercepted, and precise details were then misused to shoot at approaching rescue helicopters.

As already mentioned in the introduction, the 9 Line Medevac Request does not apply exclusively to the use of helicopters. The RCC (Rescue Coordination Center) deploys the rescue equipment that is available and makes tactical sense. This may also include ground-based rescue equipment.

In order to ensure that these rescue resources are included, an acronym from outside the NATO manuals has proven itself in the field and has thus become part of mission preparation:

S	**Security**
E	**Exploration** (of the damaged area)
R	**Rescue** (of wounded from the damaged area)
CA	**Casualty Collection Point** (CCP)
R	**Receiving reinforcements or rescue forces** within the own security area

These are some acronyms used in Tactical Medicine. There certainly are many more, as Tactical Medicine is an integral part of the tactical-operational work of military or police units.

SUMMARY:
The earlier the first indications of an incident with possible casualties are received by the RCC, the faster the appropriate rescue and support forces are deployed. These are usually on "notice-to-move" standby, which is determined individually within the operational areas: Rescue resources have a period of time X after receiving the alert until they leave their base. This varies from day to night. The earlier the first four lines of a 9 Line are sent, the faster rescue resources can be deployed. During ISAF, for example, approaching rescue helicopters received the last lines of 9 Line when they were already airborne. This saved a lot of time.

DOCUMEN-TATION

13

IN TACTICAL MEDICINE, THE TOPIC OF DOCUMENTATION IS VERY OFTEN TREATED ALMOST CARELESSLY AND SACRILEGIOUSLY.

This is usually due to the dynamic process of care in changing situations and the need for rapid evacuation in the Tactical Field Care phase. Nevertheless, documentation is extremely important during the care of an injured person or several injured people. As there are different documentation procedures, a more extensive as well as a simpler version will be discussed here.

DOCUCARD

There are many versions of attachment cards or accompanying documents for wounded people. The schematic structure of most of them is similar: a block for recording the patient data, a block for documenting the event with a date and time group, and the larger part for recording the medical measures. The timeline, which is familiar from clinical patient forms, appears on most documentation cards. There is also a stylized figure of a human body with a note to mark the location of a potential injury.

If you go through these documentation cards calmly during training, the lines and symbols that seem confusing under stress turn out to be unspectacular and logical on closer inspection. Occasionally, individual copies and versions of the cards are somewhat small, and reading them, e.g., under stress with fogged-up goggles or under low-light conditions, is rather difficult.

Some surfaces are also less user-friendly due to their texture. Water-repellent surface material is ideal, as is writing on it with waterproof felt-tip pens in blue or black. However, some cards can also be written on with a classic pencil. The variant that suits you best should be assessed in advance.

The casualty card itself should be handed over to the receiving medical personnel when the casualty is handed over. It reinforces the handover according to MIST (see Chapter 14) and gives the person taking over the opportunity to read more detailed data and

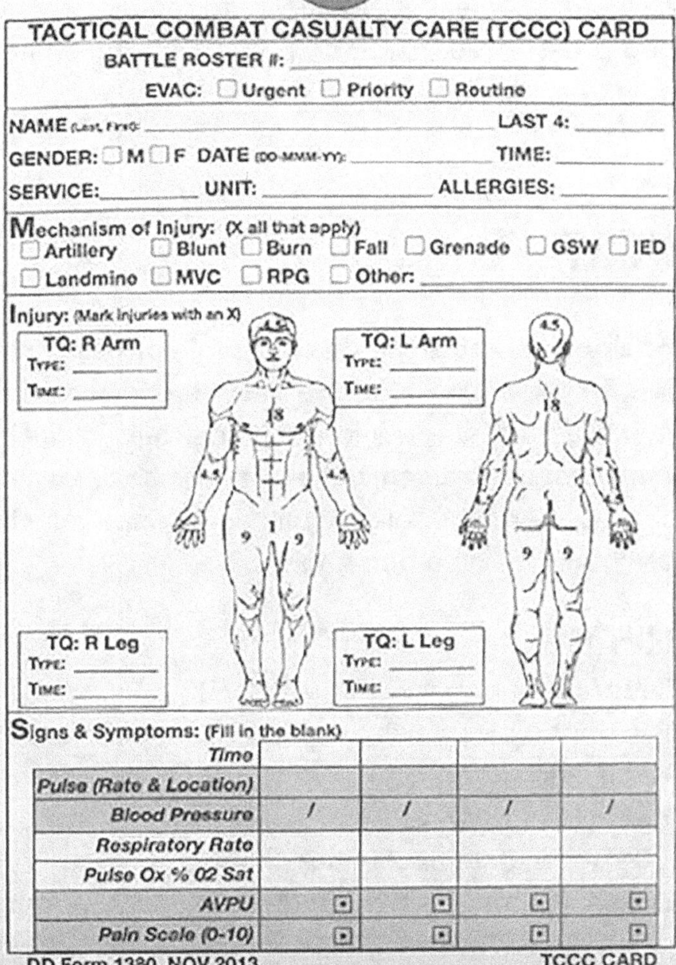

There are various casualty attachment cards, sometimes with different structures. Regardless of which card is used, it always helps with transfers of a wounded person to the receiving medical facilities.

information. Medical measures in particular, such as the administration of medication, but also the progression of vital signs, are important for follow-up care. For example, it is significant to recognize when blood pressure readings drop while the respiratory rate increases.

DOCUTAPE

If no documentation card is available or has simply been forgotten, a docutape can be created quickly. With a little preparation, this improvised means can at least transmit critical basic data on the way to follow-up care. The following is an example of what data should be on a docutape.

DOCUTAPE
- **Date/Time:** e.g., 022000 A Nov 22
- **BP:** (Blood pressure)
- **HF:** (Heart frequency)
- **RR:** (Respiratory rate)
- **TQ:** (Tourniquet application time)
- **Drugs:** (Drugs—name and quantity)

If there is no time for this form of documentation, information such as tourniquet application time **(capital T with time)** or morphine administration time **(capital M with time)** can be **written on the forehead or hand** of the injured person.

SUMMARY:

Documentation is often criminally neglected in Tactical Medicine. In addition to the transmission of sometimes essential medical information to subsequent facilities, the documentation also serves, to a certain extent, as a safeguard. If the first-aider is investigated later regarding his actions, such chronological medical records are very important. Therefore, point out the importance of documentation during training and include it as part of the exercise!

MIST REPORT

14

Tactical Medicine is usually a fast-moving, dynamic process in which changes occur abruptly. This is the case with casualty handover as well, which may have to take place while the rotor is running and under difficult conditions. There is often no room or time for chitchat or long-winded reports. If a handover is stress-free and calm, this only confirms the more dynamic rule.

Imagine, if you will, a handover from a medic to a flight medic with a running rotor and corresponding noise. This example illustrates why information must be conveyed briefly and precisely. The same applies to the handover from one medic to another at a casualty drop-off point when there is no time for detailed discussions.

The acronym **MIST** has proved its worth when it comes to passing on essential information quickly and precisely.

M echanism of injury	What has happened when? Duration of the illness?
I njury / Illness	(from head to toe)
S ymptoms	Signs of injury or vital parameters
T reatment	Measures or medication

Such a handover could sound like this:

Miller, our radio operator, stable
IED blast
Open wound on the left lower leg
Severe bleeding with pain, vital signs in normal range
Tourniquet on the left leg and morphine,
15 milligrams, ten minutes ago

As already mentioned, this is a significantly reduced version of the patient handover. In addition to this, the casualty attachment card with further information is handed over. The card can then be expanded, continued, and passed on again by the staff taking over the patient. This way, there is no information loss.

If everyone involved has more time and there are no disruptive environmental influences, the MIST report can, of course, be significantly expanded, and there can be a detailed handover. In such situations, it is also advisable to briefly inspect the affected areas of the body.

SUMMARY:

Patient handover is a sensitive interface between two levels of care, often involving the use of a transport system. To ensure that as little information as possible is lost about the patient or the measures taken, it is advisable to use tried-and-tested handover procedures. These procedures should also be included in the exercise! For example, a training situation can be resolved with a handover to the instructor in accordance with MIST.

CASEVAC / MEDEVAC 15

Similar to the 9 Line reporting scheme (see Chapter 12), these two terms are often misunderstood to always refer to airborne rescue equipment, i.e., helicopters. **This is not the case.** CASEVAC and MEDEVAC are procedures and quality designations for the evacuation of wounded personnel, usually in the Tactical Evacuation Care phase. Of course, a patient evacuation can also take place in another phase of TCCC within the framework of tactical considerations or within the framework of free capacities (or resources). Which means of rescue is used or is available depends on many factors and circumstances.

In the **CASEVAC (CASualty EVACuation)** procedure, the means of transport used does not have any medical or paramedic equipment, materials, or personnel qualifications. It is possible, for example, that ground forces request a rescue helicopter, but then a CH-47 Chinook transport helicopter lands at the point of injury (POI) on its return flight from a personnel or material transport. This helicopter may simply have been the most readily available means of transport. It is therefore the most suitable means of rescue in terms of time and space calculations. The decision as to what is assigned is made by area-wide control and coordination centers.

It is now up to the responsible forces at this landing zone to decide to what extent they will weaken their own medical forces in order to provide support for this transport, if necessary. This decision is made by the tactical leader, considering the available medical personnel. Could it mean that an ongoing operation would have to be aborted due to the weakening of his own high-value resources?

It often happens that such decisions are only discussed when the rescue vehicle has already arrived, as a different overview of the situation may have prevailed beforehand.

The **MEDEVAC (MEDical EVACuation)** procedure is the ideal case of a medical evacuation phase. Once requested and assigned, the rescue equipment arrives at the scene of the incident, possibly carrying the requested additional equipment and also replacements for used medical supplies. Such a request for medical consumables, known as a "speedball," can be included in the 9 Line report. In operational contingents, service regulations regulate such resupply procedures. Ready-made packages containing essential medical supplies are regularly available at the relevant operations centers. Not all MEDEVAC rescue equipment is of the same quality or distributed in the same way. NATO regulations, such as the NATO JOINT MEDICAL DOCTRINE, set out the common principles, but it remains a national responsibility to upgrade these minimum requirements. This also applies to the rescue equipment used. There are sometimes considerable differences. Not all rescue equipment is equalized, not even within NATO. At organizational levels such as the United Nations, these differences are sometimes even more serious.

SUMMARY:
Qualified help is not to be expected from everything that is simply called MEDEVAC. It actually depends on where and with which partner organizations or nationalities cooperation takes place. In some cases, the differences are massive and force those involved to make individual decisions for the benefit of the patient but also in the interests of the overall mission. Not everyone is aware of this, and it needs to be stressed, especially when working in the extended spectrum.

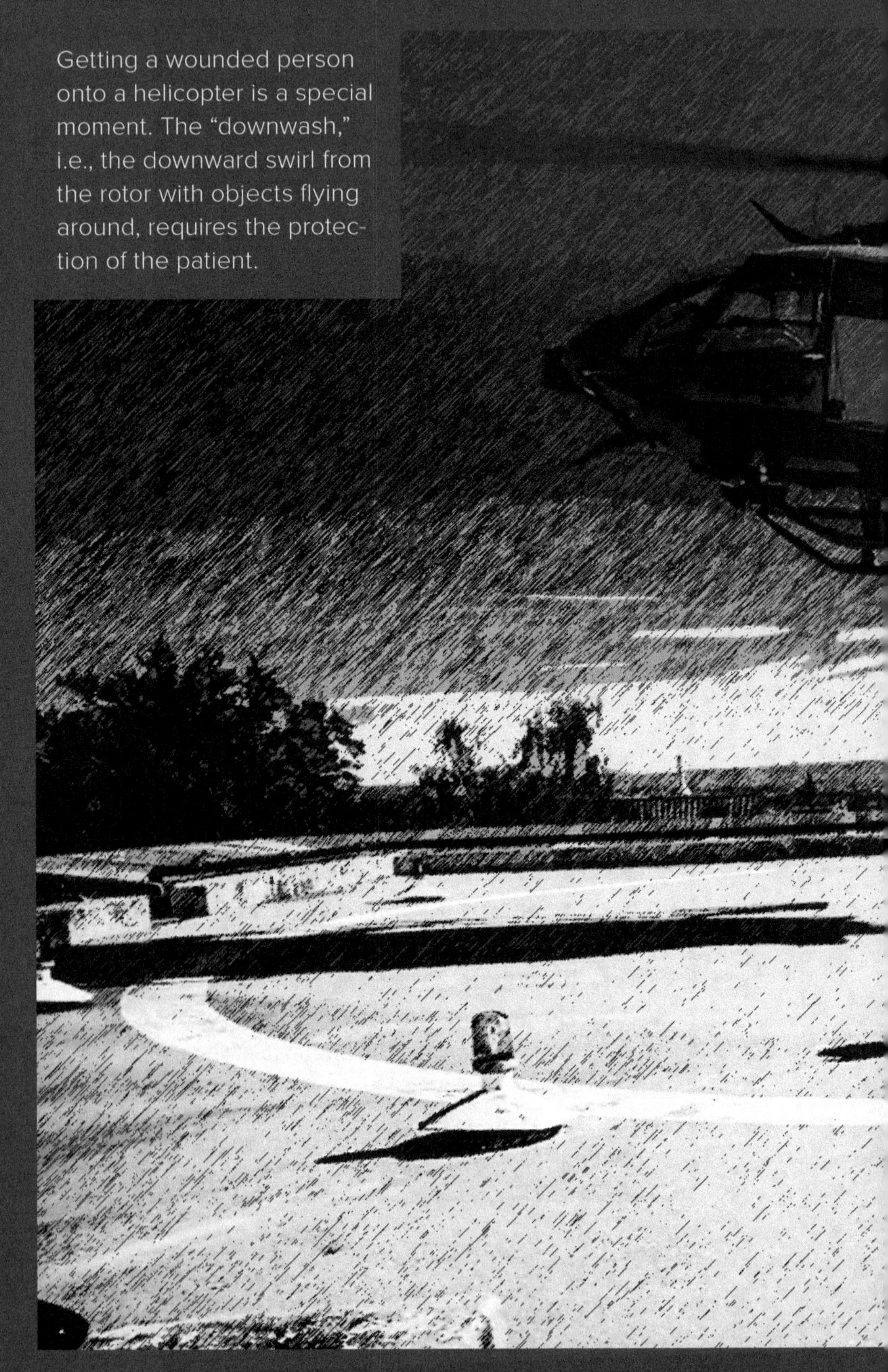

Getting a wounded person onto a helicopter is a special moment. The "downwash," i.e., the downward swirl from the rotor with objects flying around, requires the protection of the patient.

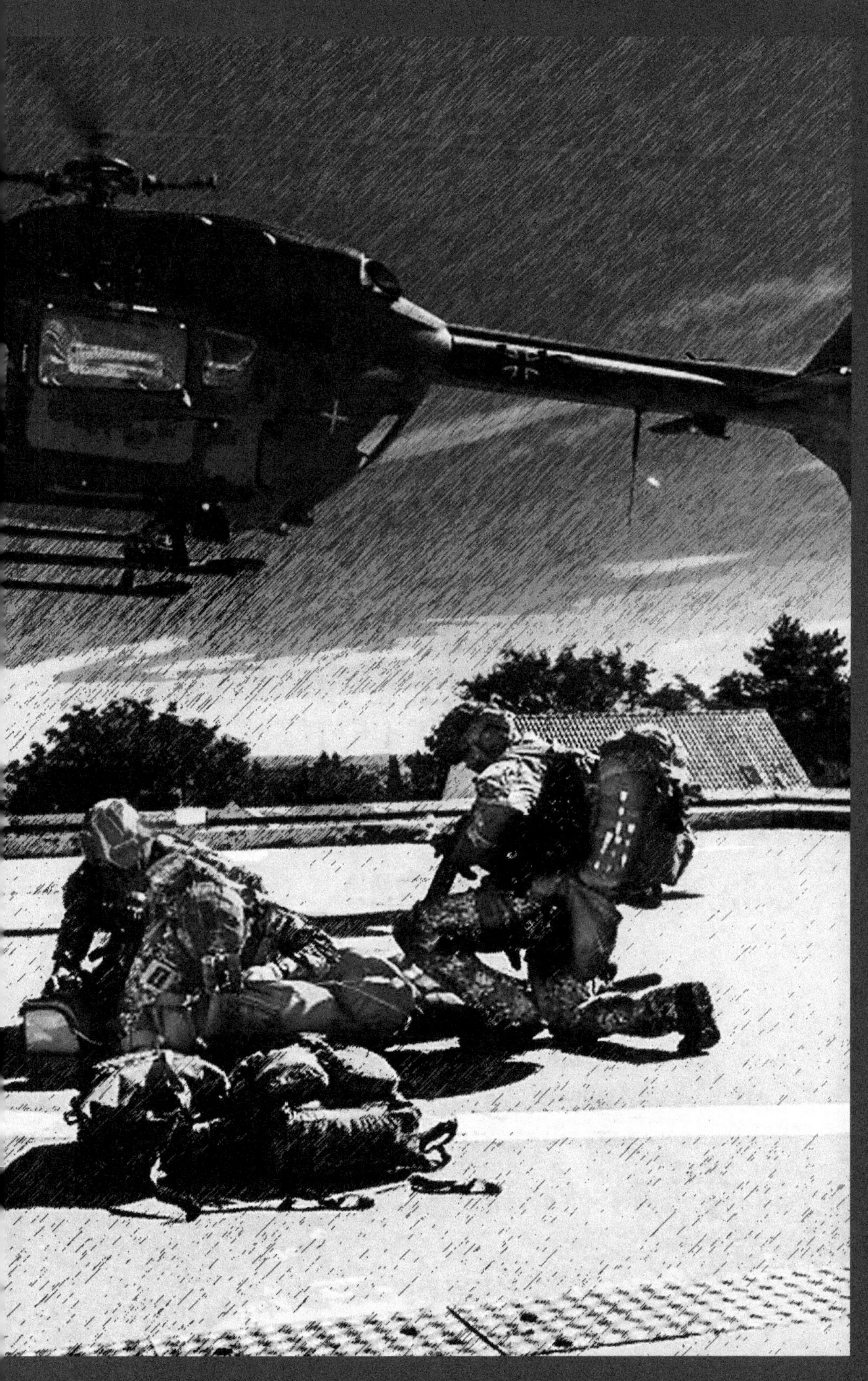

HELICOPTER LANDING ZONE 16

THE USE OF HELICOPTERS IN CASEVAC AND, ABOVE ALL, MEDEVAC OPERATIONS HAS MADE A SIGNIFICANT CONTRIBUTION TO REDUCING THE MORTALITY RATE OF THE WOUNDED ON THE BATTLEFIELD AND IN MANY OTHER EMERGENCY SITUATIONS.

There is hardly a mountain rescue mission in which not at least one attempt is made to deploy a helicopter (rotary-wing aircraft).

However, to ensure that this high-quality rescue tool can be used efficiently, ground and air rescue teams must work closely together. This also includes the preparation of a suitable landing zone (LZ).

GENERAL CONDITIONS FOR A HELICOPTER LZ

Helicopter model	Dimensions in meters
CH-53	80 × 80
CH-47	80 × 80
Super Puma	80 × 80
Mi-8	80 × 80
NH90	80 × 80
UH-1 D	50 × 50
UH-60	50 × 50
EC135/145	50 × 50

Besides that, attention should be paid to the following surface conditions:

▶ maximum gradient of 30 degrees;
▶ firm ground, test load-bearing capacity using a vehicle. If a vehicle does not sink in, a helicopter can land (for an emergency solution, carry out this test with a person sitting on your shoulders);
▶ fix loose objects—do not lay out cloths without fixing them;

▶ avoid dusty areas if possible
(downwash with brownout);
▶ avoid snow surfaces if possible
(downwash with whiteout);
▶ avoid obstacles in the direction of approach
(trees, utility poles, etc.);
▶ land against the wind; set up a windsock if
necessary.

When the helicopter is approaching, the agreed-up-on marking material (9 Line, Line 7) should be used and the signaller should be positioned in such a way that he **is stable** and **does not impede the landing helicopter.** This person should also know the correct direction signs.

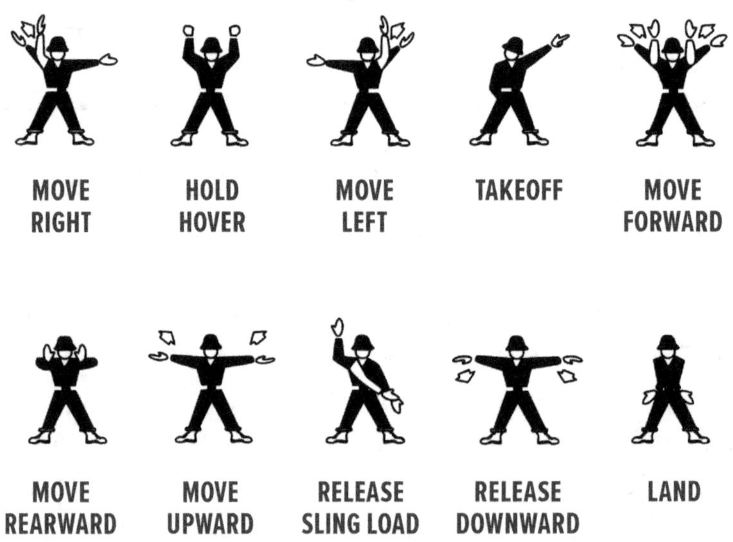

Once the helicopter has landed, make sure that the aircraft crew waves for you to approach, and only then **walk toward the helicopter from the front**; do not run, and pay attention to the rotor. The rotor can tilt dangerously low if the landing zone is inclined or sloping. If the helicopter turns off the rotor, **wait until it comes to a standstill.**

Cold loading	Rotor is stopped for loading
Hot loading	Rotor turns during loading

Preparing a landing zone is a particular challenge, especially at night or when view is limited. Below is a graphic representation of what an illuminated landing zone might look like (see sketch on the next page).

For fixed-wing aircraft like the Cessna 172 Skyhawk other conditions apply, especially with regard to the length of the landing zone. Special attention must also be paid to the necessary width. **The minimum is eleven meters.**

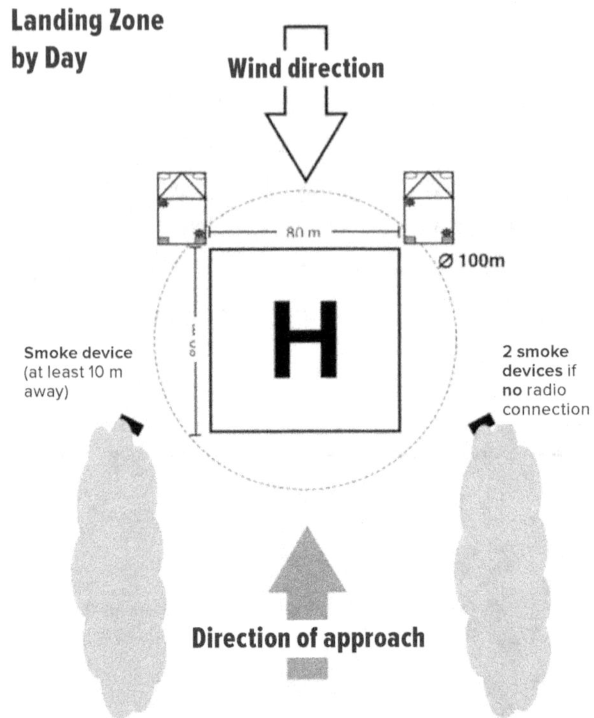

During the day and
at night, always pay
attention to

- ▶ wind direction
- ▶ obstacles
- ▶ ground gradient
- ▶ ground conditions

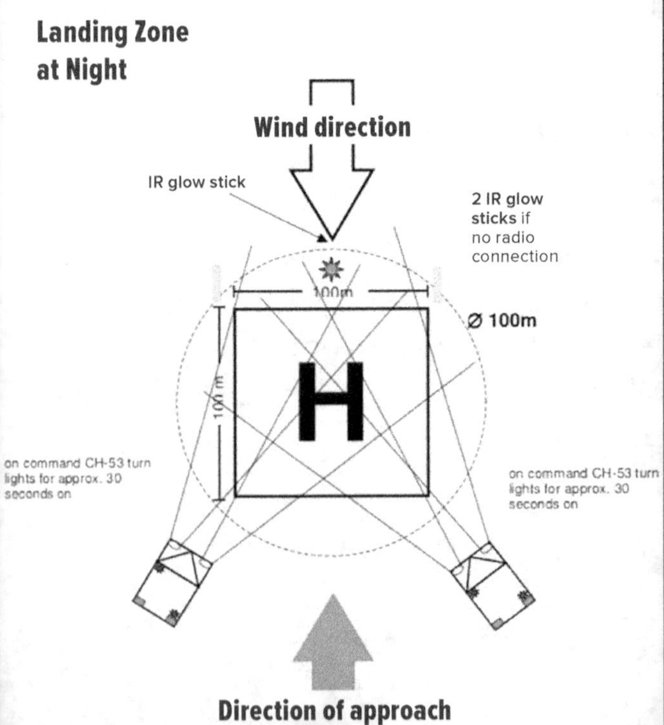

SUMMARY:
Working with an airplane or helicopter is always a very special situation that requires maximum concentration. Aircraft crews must be able to rely on the personnel supporting them on the ground, especially in adverse conditions. A mission involving such rescue equipment is not over until the helicopter or aircraft has taken off and is on its way to the destination airport or hospital. Until then, it is important to work together as a team.

LOW-LIGHT CONDITIONS

17

WAR OR MILITARY OPERATIONS OFTEN TAKE PLACE AT NIGHT OR IN THE DARK. UNFORTU-NATELY, RESCUE OPERATIONS FREQUENTLY CONTINUE INTO THE NIGHT OR EVEN BEYOND.

It is therefore essential to consider **low-light** or **no-light conditions** when preparing medical care. Anyone who only knows and is able to work in full-light mode will quickly sink into chaos in such special situations.

But how can you prepare yourself and, above all, your equipment for sub-par lighting conditions? Here are a few tips to help you handle this challenge more easily:

▶ **Get to actually know your material; get to know it fully in the light!**

▶ **Practice finding things blindfolded!**

▶ **Sort the individual items by system, for example according to cABCDE!**

▶ **Mark important items with reflective tape!**

▶ **Keep the variety of materials manageable; less is usually more!**

▶ **Secure sharp objects against accidental injury!**

▶ **Use glow sticks with a weak light effect, possibly still in the packaging with a viewing window, to illuminate specific areas!**

▶ **Learn to work under sight and light protection (tent/tarp)!**

▶ **Try to use a light-protected room whenever possible and install light barriers (e.g., overlapping blankets)!**

▶ **Where open light is necessary, use weak light sources (blue, red, or green)!**

There are certainly many other ways of working under such conditions.

The use of residual light amplifiers or night vision devices is another way to improve the situation. Often, such devices of older design or cheaper price categories only allow 2D work, i.e., there is no depth of focus. This has the effect that when moving around in the field, for example, holes are only seen as dark spots, and accessing a vein is more difficult as distances can hardly be seen and must be felt instead. The outstretched index finger can help here: **<u>Guide the needle tip along the finger to the puncture site carefully. As I said, this should, of course, be practiced, like so many other things</u>**.

SUMMARY:

A lack of light sources is a limitation that can be handled and mastered if you have practiced these special situations in advance. Professional rescuers will always incorporate the appropriate procedure into their training scenarios, as such a situation can arise more quickly than you think. Always train for the worst case; then you are prepared and will not be surprised by the circumstances. Material preparation is also part of medical planning. If you already know in advance that a rescue or search operation will last beyond daylight hours, it is almost criminally reckless not to prepare for low-light conditions.

PROLONGED FIELD CARE / PROLONGED CASUALTY CARE — 18

FOR A FEW YEARS NOW, THE WORKING TERM PROLONGED FIELD CARE [PFC], MORE RECENTLY CHANGED TO PROLONGED CASUALTY CARE [PCC], HAS BEEN USED IN CONNECTION WITH TACTICAL MEDICINE.

This phase is often erroneously referred to as the 4th phase of Tactical Combat Casualty Care (TCCC), as a kind of supplement to the Evacuation Care phase. However, this is wrong. PFC/PCC is a separate care phase that arose due to the need to provide high-quality care to injured or ill patients without access to short and functioning rescue chains or existing medical infrastructure.

For this reason, American combat medics devised a concept based on a **graduated treatment** approach. The first distinction is as follows:

▶ RUCK—TRUCK—HOUSE—PLANE

This means: treatment of the casualty
- ▶ out of the **rucksack**,
- ▶ in a **vehicle**,
- ▶ in a **building**
- ▶ or during an **evacuation**.

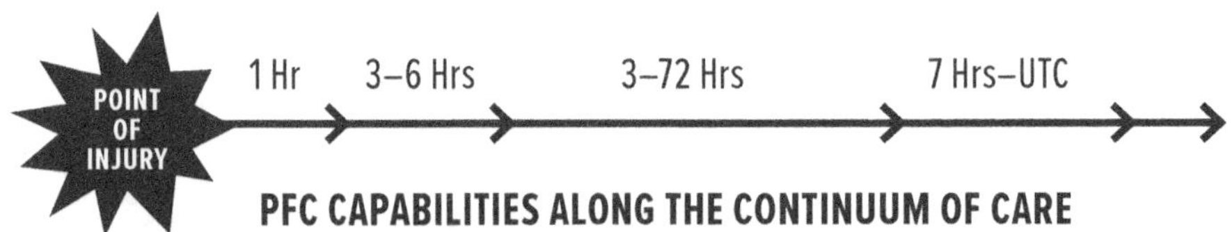

TCCC („Ruck") 1 Hr

CASEVAC („Truck") 3–6 Hrs

PATIENT HOLD („House") 3–72 Hrs

MEDEVAC („Plane") 7 Hrs–UTC

The next distinction is defined in terms of quality differences:

► GOOD / MINIMUM—BETTER—BEST

This triad depends on many factors:
- ► level of training of the rescuer(s);
- ► equipment of the rescuer(s);
- ► practical skills in the care of different patient patterns;
- ► practical skills in handling the respective materials.

In more detail, this distinction offers the possibility of evaluating personnel deployed in a care setting on the basis of not only their **basic knowledge** but also their **actual skills** and **routine**, based on **the materials available**. For example, a doctor has a high level of background knowledge but no actual specialization to perform a tracheotomy. However, the assisting medic, with additional specialist training, would be able to successfully perform this procedure based on recent repetitive drills with improvised materials.

However, in order to have qualified PFC personnel available for special areas of operation (that are usually away from the infrastructure required for regular rescue), an overview of the **basic skills** that every member of such a team should have has been compiled. This skill list comprises ten elementary subject areas, each with seven sublevels in the qualitative version:

►

10 ESSENTIAL PFC CAPABILITIES

	1. Monitoring	2. Resuscitate	3. Ventilate and oxygenate	4. Control the airways	
MINIMUM	BP Cuff, stethoscope, Pulse Ox, Foley	Fresh whole blood kit	Bag-valve-mask with PEEP Valve	Awake Ketamine Cric	
BETTER	Capnometry	2-3 cases of LR for burn resus	O_2 Concentrator	Long duration sedation	
BEST	Vital signs monitor	PRBS, FFP, type-specific donors	Portable ventilator	Proficient in rapid sequence intubation	
RUCK	Pulse Ox, head lamp	1 FWB Kit per man, 2 250cc bags NS	BVM with peep valve	Cric Kit, LMA/SGA, Lidocaine and Ketamine IM	
TRUCK	BP Cuff, stethoscope, capnometry, small monitor	Casre LR, additional vampire recipient Kits, 3% Saline	SAVent or SAVE 2	RSI, LMA/SGA, CricKit, Ketamine bag IV	
HOUSE	Add defibrillation	2 additional cases LR, Case NS, additional 3% Saline	Impact vent and O_2 bottle	All of above Add Benzo if not available for truck	
PLANE	All of above	All of above	Impact vent on O_2	All of above, calculate for flight and double	

5. Sedation and Analgesia	6. Physical Exam and Diagnostics	7. Nursing and hygiene	8. Surgical Interventions	9. Telemedical Consult	10. Package and Prepare for flight
Opiate analgesics titrated through IV	Physical exam without advanced	Clean, warm, dry, padded, catheterized	Chest tube, cric	Make comms, present patient and key vitals	Be familiar with stressors of flight
Sedation with Ketamine/option of Midazolam	Ultrasound and point of care labs	Bed debride-ment, washout NG/OG	Fasciotomy, debridement, amputation	Add labs and ultrasound video	Trained in critical care transport
Educated and practiced multi-drug sedation	Experienced and trained in above	Experienced in all nursing care concerns	Trained and experienced in above	Real time video conference	Experienced in critical care transport
Fentanyl TML, Perc PO, Ketamin IM/IV	Urinalysis test strips, fluoresce-in strips	Compact foley kit, sterile kerlix, litter padding	Cric, 10g Needle D, Scalpel	Cell phone and call sheet	Have checklist available
Ketamine IV with Midazolam	Blood tubes to drop off at labs on the way	Padded litter, NG	Sterile chest tube kit with drapes	Cell phone and call sheet, sat phone, radio	Checklist plus flight evac kit
Same as above	Blood tubes to drop off at local clinic	Real mattress with head elevated, nursing care kit, sleeping bag	Sterile surgical kit with drapes, gowns and scrub soap	Secure comms, email	Extensive evac kit
of above, cal-culate for flight and double		Padded litter, sleeping bag	10g needle D, chest tube kit, CricKit	Through aircraft	All of above

In the event of a need for PFC care, more extensive protocols and schemes are used. The possibility of telemedicine support is also strongly favored.

For example, the familiar MARCH scheme is extended to **MARCH2H3 – PAWS-L**:

M	Massive Haemorrhage Control (MASCAL)
A	Airways
R	Respiration
C	Circulation
C	Communication
H	Hypothermia—Hyperthermia
H	Head injuries
P	Pain control
A	Antibiotics
W	Wounds (nursing plus burns)
S	Splinting
L	Logistics

SUMMARY:

Prolonged Field Care or Prolonged Casualty Care is a good way of providing the best possible treatment for sick or injured persons, even away from functioning rescue chains, by means of an adapted (and above all honest) consideration of medical capabilities. In the run-up to such deployment options, the basics of PFC/PCC should be included in the preparation. However, the aim is always to avoid this phase through a timely and effective evacuation.

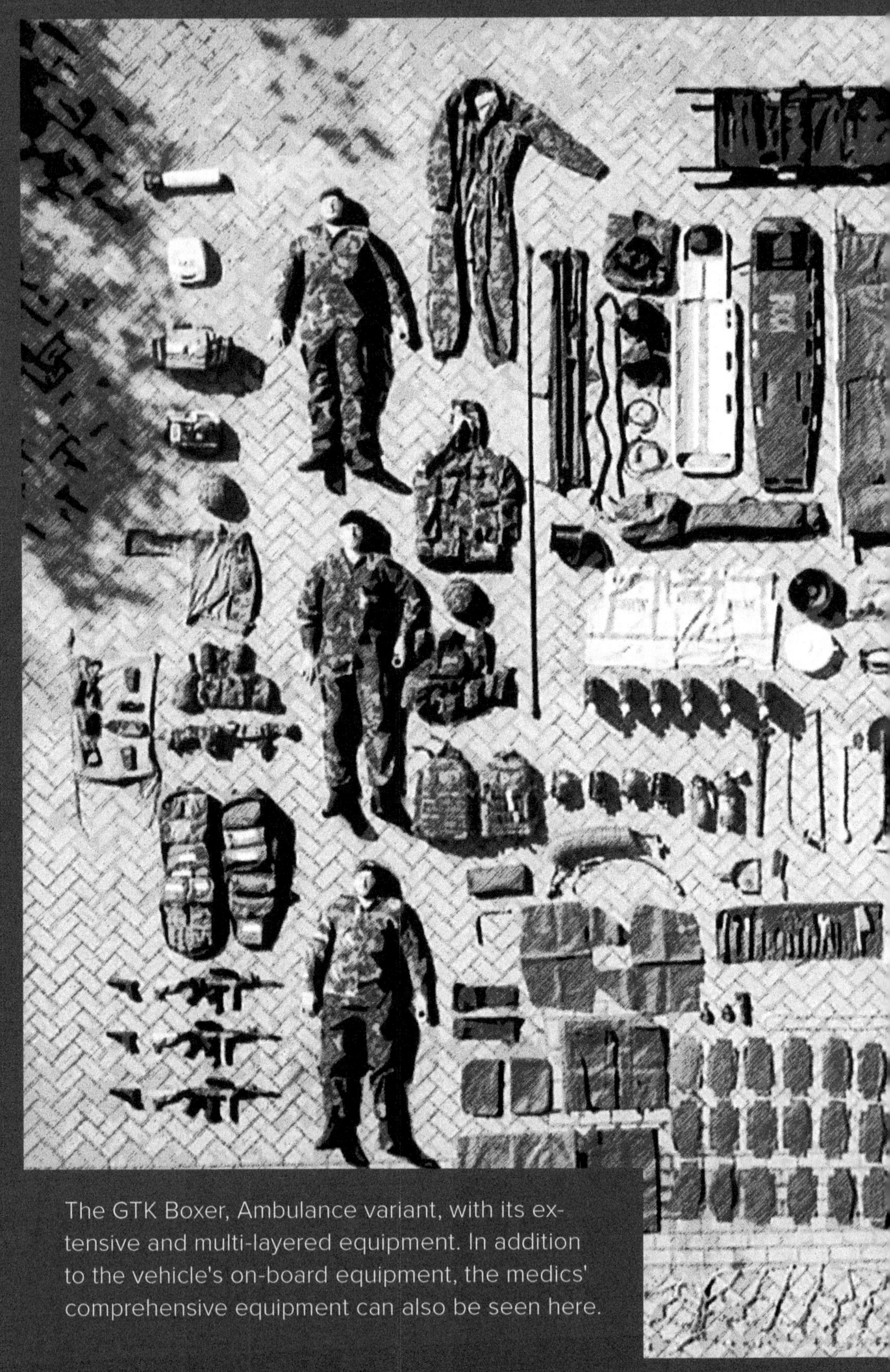

The GTK Boxer, Ambulance variant, with its extensive and multi-layered equipment. In addition to the vehicle's on-board equipment, the medics' comprehensive equipment can also be seen here.

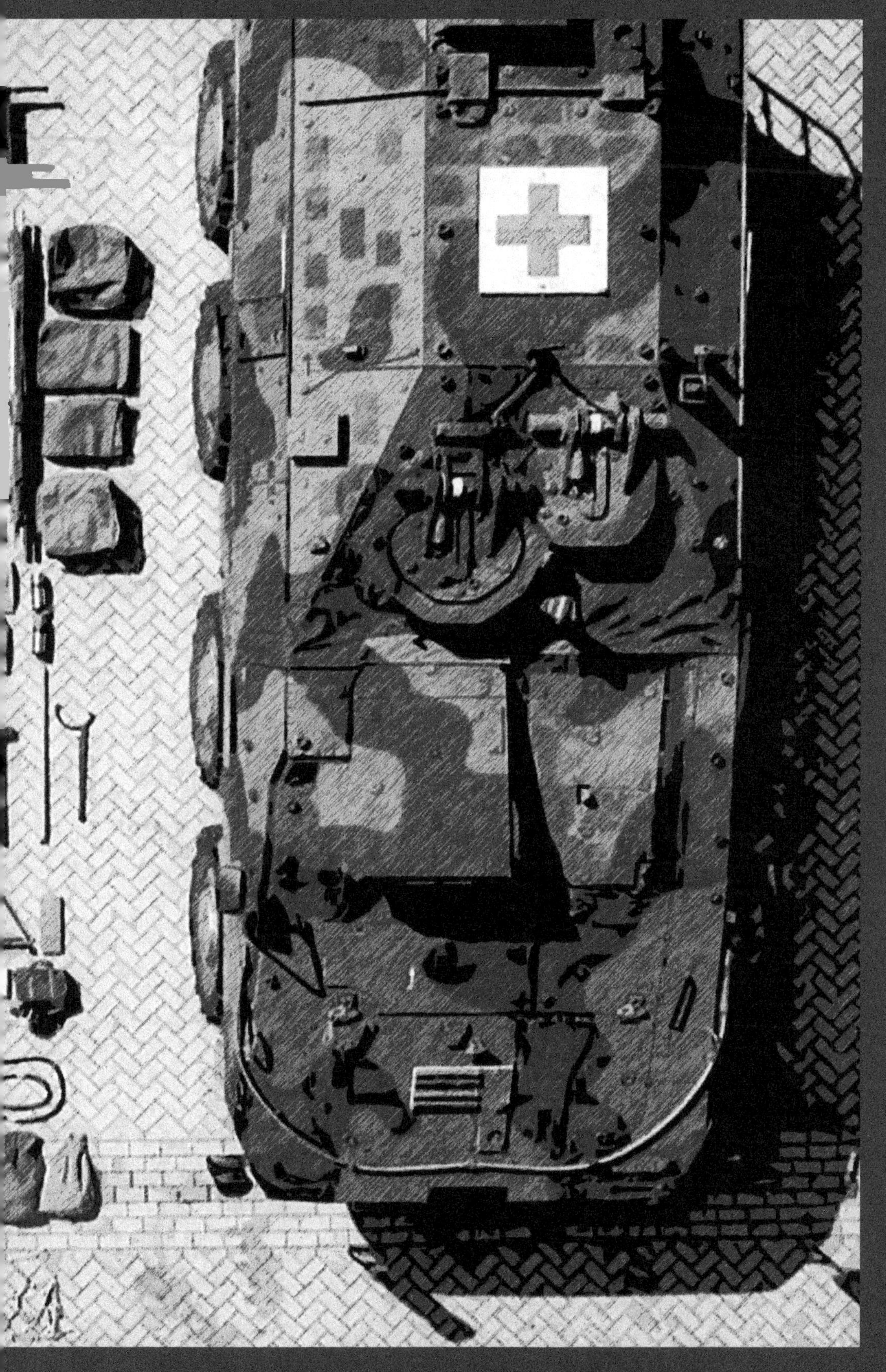

THE TEN COMMANDMENTS OF TACTICAL MEDICINE 19

1. PREPARE DILIGENTLY FOR YOUR MISSION.

Continuous learning and ongoing education in the special field, but also in related areas, is a lifelong task for someone who wants to work within Tactical Medicine at a high level.

2. BE A GOOD TEAM PLAYER, BUT ALSO BE PREPARED TO WORK ALONE.

Working together as a team and putting your own ego aside are prerequisites for successful missions. Nevertheless, everyone should also be able to complete their assignment on their own. Waiting for help from others to be able to function is often not helpful. You are frequently forced to take the initiative and make a decision on your own, if necessary.

3. ALWAYS LOOK BEYOND YOUR OWN NOSE WHEN PREPARING.

Learn from the skills of others inside and outside your team. If you don't ask, you won't get an answer. An answer that could perhaps help overcome an emergency situation. At the same time, it helps to develop a better understanding of other people's areas of work.

4. GET SUPPORT IN BEFORE IT'S TOO LATE.

Excessive ego or cowardice regularly leads to disaster. Ask for help and support in good time before you can no longer find a way out, and all that remains in the end is damage limitation. Asking questions shows strength, not weakness.

5. KNOW YOUR MATERIAL AS WELL AS YOUR EQUIPMENT.

Dangerous half-knowledge provides a false sense of security and can quickly lead you to the limits of your own safety in an emergency. Mastering something means constantly handling it in order to have reserves, even in extreme situations. If you are already at the limit when handling your equipment, you will fail under pressure.

6. CONSIDER YOURSELF AND YOUR PATIENT IMPORTANT, BUT NOT ALL-IMPORTANT.

Tactical Medicine is first and foremost a team mission, followed by the need to look after the individual. Always keep this in mind, and be aware that you are not always a top priority.

7. MEDICAL PLANNING ACCOUNTS FOR 80% OF SUCCESSFUL CARE.

Many things that should be taken for granted in an emergency situation can easily be planned or determined in peace. This includes not only equipment but also medical facilities along the marching route. Don't rely on old, possibly out-dated, documents from your predecessors.

8. LEARN TO IMPROVISE.

Off-label uses and the ability to improvise can considerably expand your own material re-sources. If you only think stubbornly within your own scheme, you can quickly reach your limits.

9. TACTICS DETERMINE MEDICINE, SO BE AWARE OF THIS.

This awareness is often unfamiliar territory for medical staff in particular. Cues such as "no play," which we are familiar with from training scenarios, regularly don't help in a real emergency. In most cases, medical personnel also lack an overview of the whole situation. Therefore, listen to and believe the instructions of the tactical leader. This does not mean that you cannot make a professional recommendation or request.

10. KEEP YOURSELF PHYSICALLY FIT.

The physical fitness of many everyday rescuers leaves a lot to be desired. Everyone can imagine for themselves what this performance can look like when transporting injured people over longer distances with makeshift equipment, for example. Anyone who reaches their physical limits while climbing three flights of stairs certainly has no place in tactical medicine.

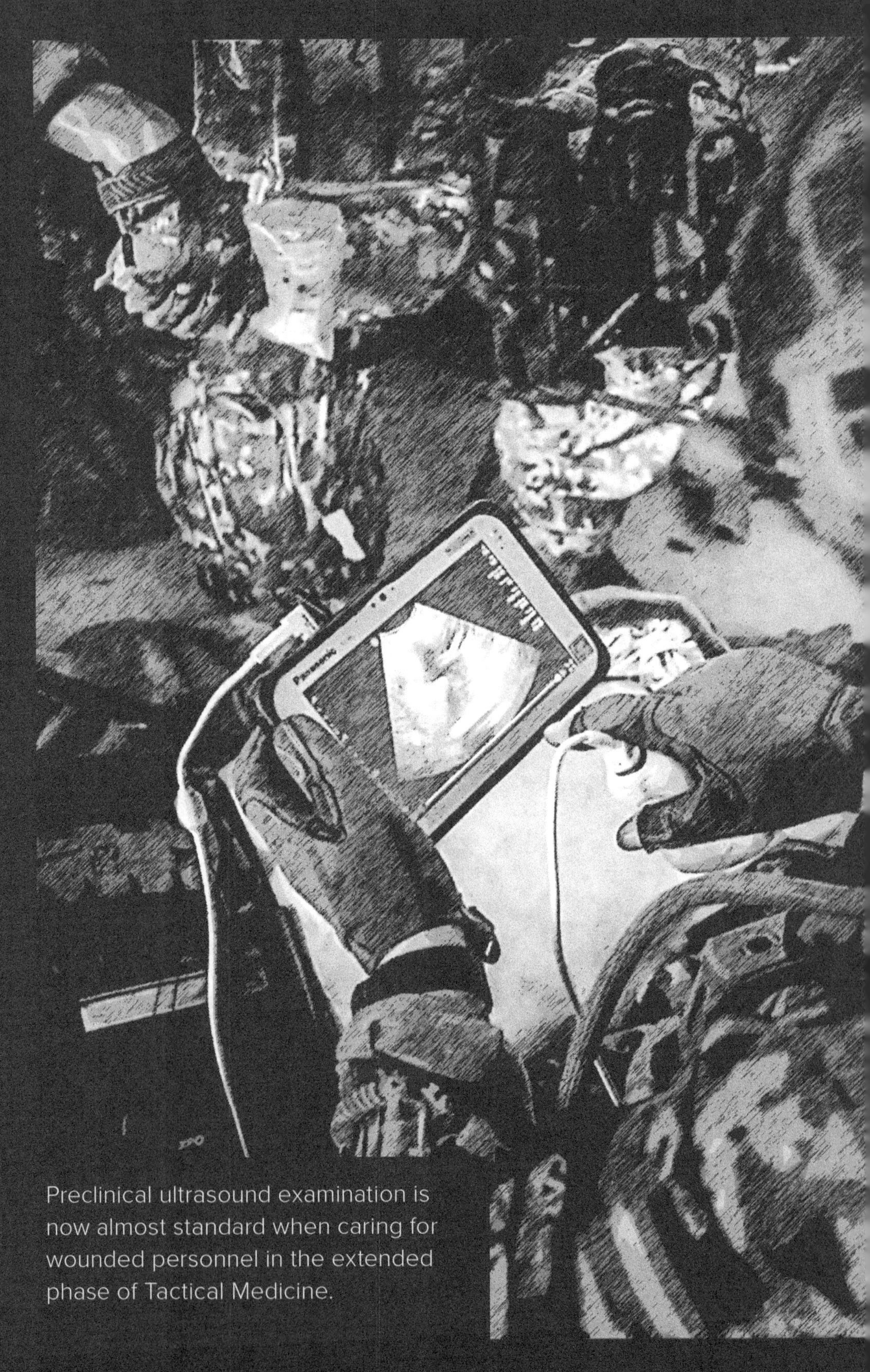

Preclinical ultrasound examination is now almost standard when caring for wounded personnel in the extended phase of Tactical Medicine.

TACTICAL MEDICINE IS POPULAR AND SEEMS TO BE THE ONLY MEANS OF CHOICE AND THE LAST RESORT IN MANY AREAS.

It is very often forgotten that although individual elements of Tactical Medicine can be used in many areas, not everything is needed across the board.

After creating this awareness, the next step is to take a reflective look at your own equipment. Here, too, it seems to me that very frequently, the target has been clearly overshot. Work areas that appear completely overloaded, to an almost grotesque degree, and that seem to follow a certain cult. Here, too, it should be noted that less is sometimes more. Tactical Black seems to be the color of the season for many at the moment.

A final aspect of Tactical Medicine concerns the choice of training. Not everything called TCCC/TECC, for example, is actually TCCC/TECC in the end. There's a lot of window-dressing and gimmickry going on in the current training scene. Everyone seems to want to secure a piece of the pie. Unfortunately, applicants interested in such training often lack a comparative tool when choosing their courses, and more or less well-done advertising pages disguise actual shortcomings. In the end, a lot of money and energy are regularly wasted, and dangerous half-knowledge is conveyed. Sometimes you want to shout out loud: "Cobbler, stick to your last!" Knowledge of emergency services and tactical operational training do not make an instructor of Tactical Medicine. There must be an overall understanding. There is no other explanation for the frequently observed discussions with so-called experts about where to apply tourniquets. Unfortunately, this is just one example of many that shows the extent to which standard emergency medical services and Tactical Medicine are mixed up and freely interpreted.

Tactical Medicine is not a competitor to conventional procedures of standard rescue or maximum care individual medicine, which have developed and proven themselves over the years. Tactical Medicine closes a gap within a rescue chain and starts where previous procedures offer no options for action due to various causes and factors.

FURTHER READING

+ TACTICAL COMBAT CASUALTY CARE HANDBOOK

This U.S. Army TCCC handbook was created for soldiers and medical personnel to practice medical treatment from point of injury to evacuation.

Department of Defense
Tactical Combat Casualty Care Handbook
Department of Defense, 133 pages, paperback,
5th edition 2023

+ SPECIAL OPERATIONS FORCES MEDICAL HANDBOOK

The newest edition of the Special Operations Forces Medical Handbook is perfect and practical for both soldiers and civilians. Nearly 140 comprehensive illustrations show the proper techniques for medical care, from basic first-aid and orthopedics to instructions for emergency war surgery and even veterinary medicine. Questions are listed so that the medic can obtain an accurate patient history and perform a complete physical examination. Diagnoses are made easier with information on the distinctive features of each illness. This straightforward manual is sure to assist any reader faced with a medical issue or emergency.

Department of Defense
Special Operations Forces Medical Handbook
Department of Defense, 676 pages, 2016

+ RANGER MEDIC HANDBOOK

The official U.S. Army special forces first-aid and medical emergency treatment of head injuries, burns, anaphylactic shock, and much more.

Rangers value honor and reputation more than their lives, and as such will attempt to lay down their own lives in defense of their comrades. The Ranger Medic will do no less. Historically in warfare, the majority of all combat deaths have occurred prior to a casualty ever receiving advanced trauma management. Ranger leaders can significantly reduce the number of Rangers who die of wounds sustained in combat by simply targeting optimal medical capability in close proximity to the point of wounding. Directing casualty response management and evacuation is a Ranger leader task; ensuring technical medical competence is a Ranger Medic task.

Department of Defense
150 pages, 2016

+ PARARESCUE MEDICAL OPERATIONS (PJ MED)

The Pararescue Medical Operations Handbook forms the basis of medical practice during Rescue Operations and training mishaps for USAF Pararescuemen (PJs).

This revised handbook includes an outline of the principles of PJ medicine and the patient assessment checklist. This approach to patients is slightly modified from traditional primary and secondary surveys to reflect a more efficient and comprehensive approach to combat trauma based on PJ experience and data from Overseas Contingency Operations. This handbook includes portions of the Tactical Combat Casualty Care (TCCC) guidelines and the ATP Tactical Medical Emergency Protocols (TMEPS) pertaining to Pararescue. These protocols have are to suit the PJ mission. The goal remains to all PJs work to a single standard. The section on prolonged care has been modified and expanded based on PJ experiences.

Pararescue Medical Operations (PJ MED)
U.S. Air Force, 441 pages, 8. Edition January 2021

+ JSOM'S ADVANCED TACTICAL PARAMEDIC PROTOCOLS [ATP-P] BOOK

The Advanced Tactical Protocols-Paramedic (ATP-P) Handbook is an essential reference tool for tactical and combat medics, SWAT team members, and medical professionals operating in austere environments. This handbook is printed on standard paper and is NOT waterproof or tearproof.

This handbook contains the 2016-2019 TMEPS TTPs, as well as the current TCCC, PCC, and cTCCC guidelines. We updated the ToC to make it more comprehensive and user-friendly.

JSOM's Advanced Tactical Paramedic Protocols
U.S. Special Operations Command, 310 pages, 11th edition 2022

+ SPECIALIST MAGAZINE

The best-known specialist magazine is the Journal of Special Operations Medicine (JSOM).

jsomonline.org

APPENDIX

- + COMBAT FIRST RESPONDER
- + IFAK
- + KNOCKOFFS AND COUNTERFEITS

COMBAT FIRST RESPONDER

In the German Federal Armed Forces, both the Army (KSK) and Navy Special Forces (KSM), as well as the Specialized Army Forces, undergo Tactical Medical training to qualify as a **Combat First Responder (CFR)**.

This is part of the basic specialist training for every member of one of these units.

CFR training is currently divided into three levels:

CFR A
(similar to a Combat Medic), duration: 6 days
- ▶ MARCH scheme
- ▶ basic anatomy
- ▶ hemostasis
- ▶ trauma care
- ▶ heat preservation
- ▶ TCCC phases
- ▶ 9 Line Medevac
- ▶ transportation methods
- ▶ documentation

CFR B

duration: 4.5 weeks

- ▶ CFR A knowledge
- ▶ advanced anatomy
- ▶ invasive measures, such as I.V. and I.O. lines
- ▶ drug administration
- ▶ advanced airway management
- ▶ prolonged casualty care
- ▶ tactical air transport with care in the helicopter

CFR C

duration: 4.5 months

- ▶ CFR B
- ▶ paramedic training
- ▶ tactical drill week

In Germany, CFR training takes place at the Special Operations Training Center in Pfullendorf. In addition to the training of German special forces, there is an international inspectorate for the training of NATO special forces at this location, the International Special Training Center (ISTC) as well. This center offers a medical course for nonmedical personnel, the NATO Special Operations Combat Medics (NSOCM) course. This course takes about five months.

- ▶ **Special Operations Training Center:**
  bit.ly/3OZA1a7
- ▶ **International Special Training Center:**
  istc-sof.org

IFAK

INDIVIDUAL FIRST AID KIT (IFAK) IS THE GENERIC TERM FOR CUSTOMIZED FIRST AID EQUIPMENT.

It is precisely the individuality concept that makes it possible for users to put together such an IFAK specifically according to their own training, the mission, and the respective environmental conditions.

The individually assembled tool kit differs significantly from common, mass-produced goods in that it is not standardized off-the-shelf and therefore usually not overloaded or incomplete. It is thus not surprising that this abbreviation has long since left the realm of special forces or specialists in general and is now also used across the entire range of possible applications.

Recently, the recommendation for an individual IFAK composition has been extended from humans to animals. There are already IFAKs prepared for the K9, i.e., the service dog, as well as for trail riding purposes. In the latter case, materials for both horse and rider are recommended to be kept in the same saddlebag. What was deemed unthinkable a short time ago has become possible thanks to the development of new materials.

Almost all IFAKs contain the following basic equipment:
- ▶ sanitary gloves
- ▶ tourniquet
- ▶ rescue blanket
- ▶ gauze and/or stretch bandage
- ▶ plaster set
- ▶ sanitizing equipment (swabs, agents)

The bag itself, especially in terms of color, size, and mount, is really a very personal decision, but functionality should always be taken into account. If you purchase an IFAK with military MOLLE loops, for example, you should then actually have a MOLLE system to hold it.

As already described, additional equipment is provided as well, depending on requirements, training, budget, and resources.

Additional items could include:
- ▶ hemostatic agents
- ▶ Wendl and/or Guedel tubes for airway management
- ▶ special equipment such as tick tongs, muzzles, tweezers, etc.

Whatever your own IFAK eventually looks like, the items included should be well-known and familiar. **This means that training in handling the material is essential.**

MY IFAK

THE INDIVIDUAL FIRST AID KIT (IFAK) IS YOUR PERSONAL RESCUE BOX, ALWAYS AT HAND.

(1) THE BOOBOO KIT
Various plasters for minor injuries.

(2) THE RESCUE BLANKET
Guarantees heat retention.

(3) GLOVES
Work with protection.

(4) PRESSURE BANDAGE
Classic Israeli bandage.

(5) LUBRICANT
But for the nose.

(6) WENDL TUBE
Keeps the nose clear.

(7) DECOMPRESSION NEEDLE
Against pneumothorax.

(8) CHEST SEAL
Against holes in the chest.

(9) COMBAT GAUZE
Stops bleeding.

ATTACHMENT CARD
For documentation.
▶ see p. 79

▶ more IFAK information: p. 124

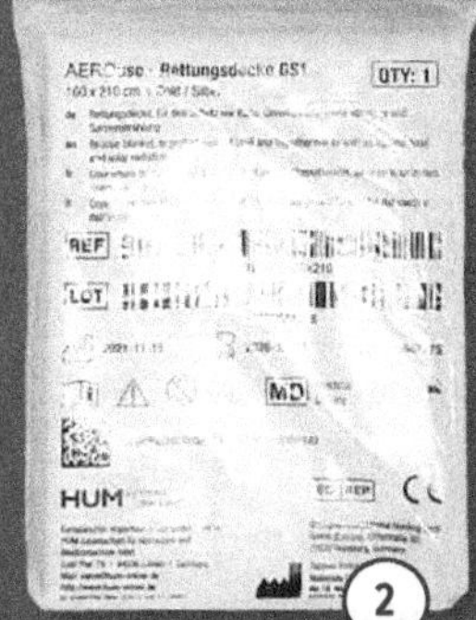
AEROuse - Rettungsdecke GS1
160 x 210 cm
QTY: 1
REF
LOT
HUM
MD

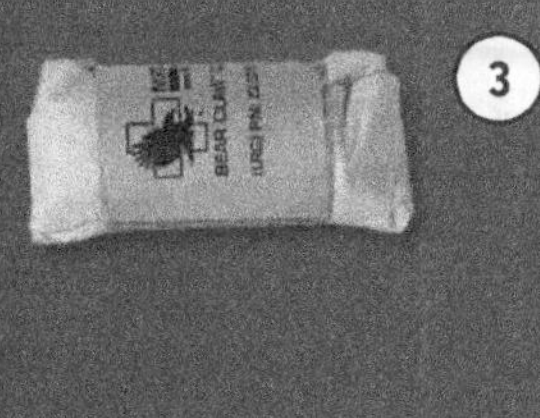
BEAR CLAW

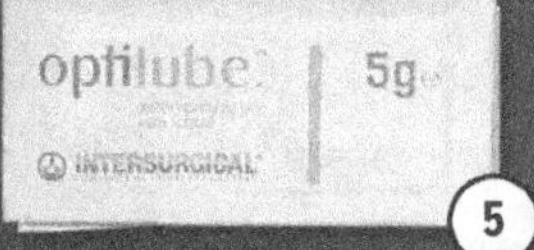

optilube
5g
INTERSURGICAL

ARS

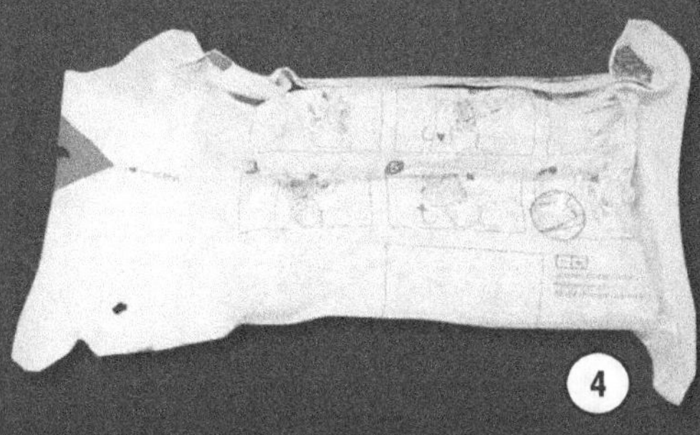

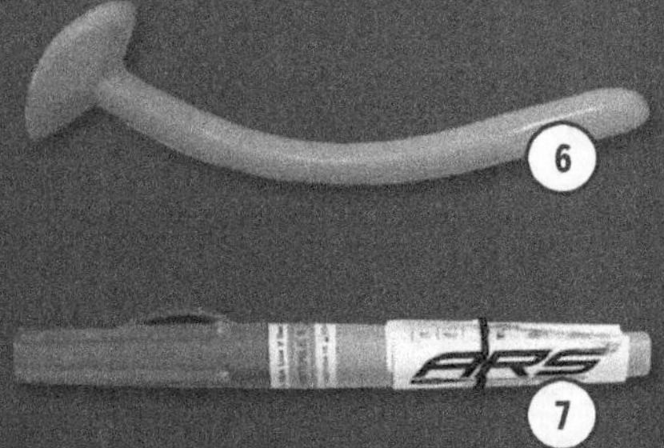

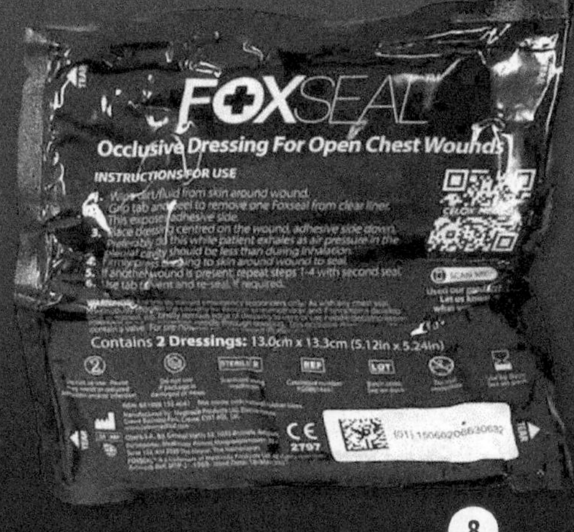
FOXSEAL
Occlusive Dressing For Open Chest Wounds
INSTRUCTIONS FOR USE
Contains 2 Dressings: 13.0cm x 13.3cm (5.12in x 5.24in)
STERILE R
REF
LOT
CE
2797

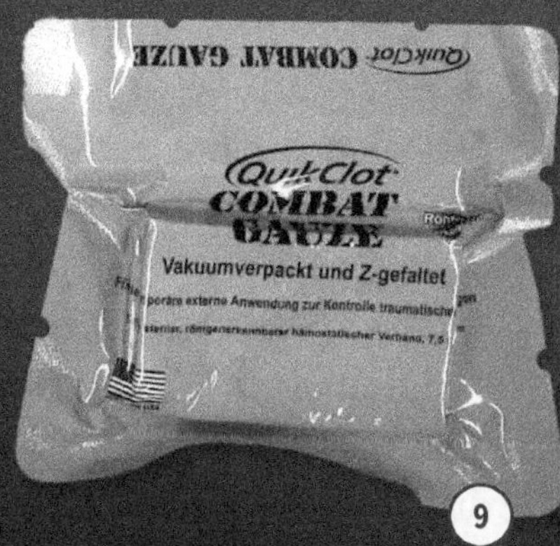
QuikClot COMBAT GAUZE
QuikClot
COMBAT
GAUZE
Vakuumverpackt und Z-gefaltet

KNOCKOFFS AND COUNTERFEITS

Who does not know the cheap products from the so-called black market, some of which are very similar to the original? We find them along the roads near the border or at bazaars, just a few hours to the south: polo shirts, handbags, or watches. Everything that ordinary people can't afford is suddenly available for a fraction of the money.

Who cares if the quality of the product then deteriorates a few weeks after the "bargain" purchase, and the item is thrown away? Somehow, many people have one or more of these souvenirs in their possession, although they at least suspect that this is not entirely legal. Many people overlook this as a supposedly trivial offense.

With the rise and nowadays massive dominance of online trading platforms, the business of knockoff products is literally booming. There seems to be almost nothing that will not be copied in the Far East and then appear on European and American markets at dumping prices. It is thus hardly surprising that the medical device industry has become a target for such dubious and illegal machinations as well.

Our aim here is to educate, protect, and ultimately even save lives. First, a few formal notes on the legal background of medical devices.

In the U.S., medical devices are regulated by the Food and Drug Administration (FDA). Information on this can be found at: **fda.gov**.

In Europe, medical devices are regulated by EU directives. In detail: EU90/385 regarding active implants, EU98/79 regarding in vitro diagnostics, and EU93/42 regarding other medical devices. Annex IX of EU93/42 also defines the following **risk classification:**

Class I: e.g., disposable syringes, plasters, or dressings; low invasiveness, no or non-critical skin contact, temporary use ≤ 60 minutes.

Class IIA: e.g., chest seals or aspirators; moderate invasiveness, short-term application ≤ 30 days, continuous or repeated use of the same product.

Class IIB: e.g., ventilators or defibrillators; increased methodological risk, systemic effects, long-term application ≥ 30 days.

Class III: e.g., heart valves or stents; high hazard potential, particularly high medical risk.

The three EU directives have been implemented nationally in each EU member state by **medical device laws**. Germany has a Medical Devices Act with 44 articles (2016 version), Austria has a Medical Devices Act with 117 articles (2015 version).

Germany also has a Medical Devices Regulation and a Medical Devices Safety Plan Regulation. In 2017, directives EU90/385 and EU93/42 were supplemented by regulation EU2017/745. By upgrading the EU directives to an EU regulation, national legal implementation is no longer necessary.

Details on legal requirements are available from the respective national controlling authority:

Germany:
bfarm.de/DE/Medizinprodukte/_node.html

Austria:
basg.gv.at/medizinprodukte/ (page 4 of 11)

In the run-up to a purchase of medical devices, it would be advisable to contact these authorities in case of uncertainties or specific questions in order to obtain a valid CE approval and, if necessary, operating instructions. So much for the legal basis.

Unfortunately, **white-collar crime** also occurs with medical devices, whether by manufacturers who do not adhere to specifications or by distributors who see profit as their main priority and therefore tread on thin legal ice. Whether this is done intentionally or in ignorance of the legal requirements is irrelevant. The spectrum ranges from gray imports that do not meet legal requirements to plagiarism and knockoff products that are clearly illegal!

The penal provisions in Germany according to the Medical Devices Act (MPG) §40, with up to three years and, in serious cases, up to five years imprisonment, show that the legislator is serious.

In addition to criminal violations of MPG, there may also be civil violations of trademark and patent laws. If a product does not yet have a valid CE approval, an approval procedure could be initiated, and the purchaser would then switch to the manufacturer or marketer.

It is evident that such a CE approval procedure is associated with significant costs, but there is no guarantee whether the product in question will be approved or not. There is a specific warning from Interpol Washington (Control No. 0-420/1-2018, File No. 2018/7564-1) that explicitly references the **purchase of counterfeit tourniquets**.

A quick glance at the prices of various offers on the Internet should usually be enough. Take, for example, the "special offer" of CAT 7s (Combat Application Tourniquets, 7th Generation) on a platform like eBay or Amazon—three pieces for €9.99.

This advice is also addressed to the authorities, in which personnel deployed for the procurement of operational or training material very often, unfortunately, look at the price first and then commit disciplinary offenses and/or criminal offenses by purchasing counterfeits.

Irrespective of the legal aspects mentioned above, the use of replica medical devices entails **high risks during deployment**.

Using a series of experiments, I have demonstrated how cheap and poor quality can make the use of such products a case of brinkmanship, or rather, a gamble with the life of the patient treated with them.

For this purpose, I purchased a CAT 7 replica from an online retailer (around €7/unit). The test series was carried out with the knowledge and approval of the regular European importer, who also provided the certified original CAT 7 (around €35/unit).

For the test, the replica was placed around a 30 cm-diameter column, pre-tensioned, and then tightened, in comparison with the original. The replica contorted and was unable to build up pressure evenly.

In sum, it is particularly important to point out the considerable

DANGER TO LIFE AND LIMB OF THE CASUALTY THROUGH THE USE OF A KNOCKOFF

In a situation where no mistakes should be made and where every rescuer blindly relies on the functionality of the material provided, failure, e.g., due to material weakness, can easily lead to the death of the wounded person. This also happens under operational conditions. We have heard from Ukraine, especially, about the failure of Chinese tourniquet clones and about paramedics who are desperately looking for original tourniquets and medical material because only these can reliably save lives.

Only the original does what is expected of it. This is something you need to be aware of when procuring medical products.

MEDICINE OUTSIDE THE COMFORT ZONE

MEDICINE OUTSIDE THE COMFORT ZONE IS THE MOTTO OF THE CAPSARIUS ACADEMY.

This includes tactical medicine, but also the influences of the environment.

The Capsarius Academy offers online courses for this purpose.

Further information can be found at:

https://elearning.capsarius-akademie.com/ kurse-taktische-medizin

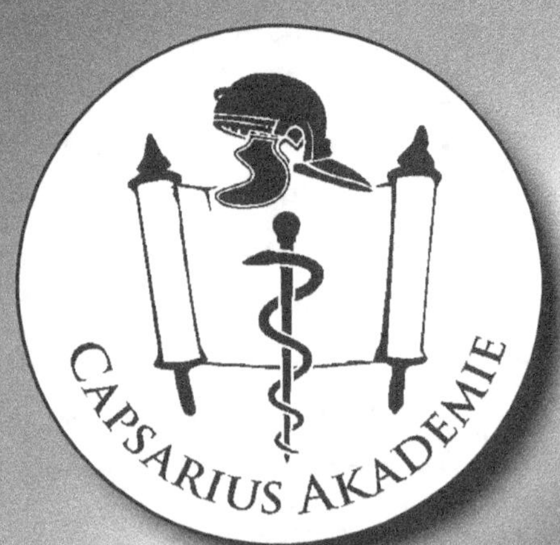

ABOUT THE AUTHOR

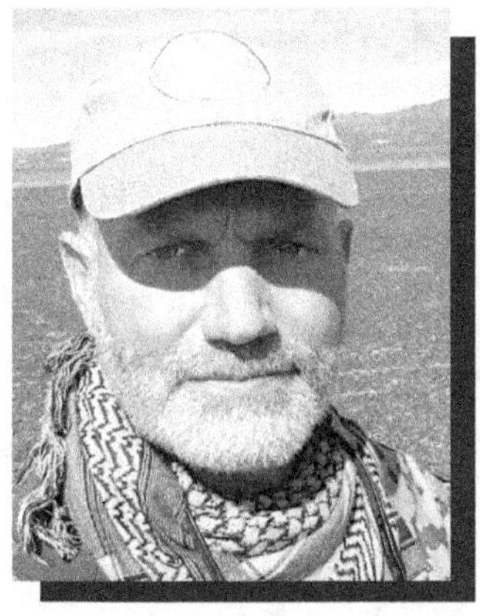

CARSTEN DOMBROWSKI

served in the German Federal Armed Forces (Bundeswehr) for many decades as a specialist instructor, expert, and lecturer on Tactical Medicine. He has been involved with TCCC in the Bundeswehr and German police from the very beginning. He himself has been deployed many times with the Bundeswehr, NATO, and the United Nations and is regarded as experienced and authentic in his approach.

After his active military service, Dombrowski founded the Capsarius Academy, which focuses on the topic of "medicine outside the comfort zone." He is also a founding member of TREMA e.V., where he was responsible for the training and further education of TREMA members for many years. As a permanent member of the editorial board of the magazine "Taktik & Medizin," he regularly publishes specialist articles. He has authored various technical books on this subject as well.

SPARTANAT
MILITARY NEWS
TACTICAL LIFE
GEAR & REVIEWS
THIS
IS OUR
WORLD ▼
ALL LINKS:
LINKTR.EE/
SPARTANAT

www.ingramcontent.com/pod-product-compliance
Lightning Source LLC
LaVergne TN
LVHW011017200726
843509LV00011B/1135